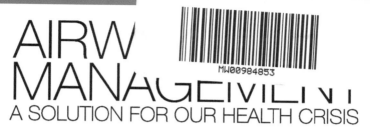

AIRW
MANAGEMENT
A SOLUTION FOR OUR HEALTH CRISIS

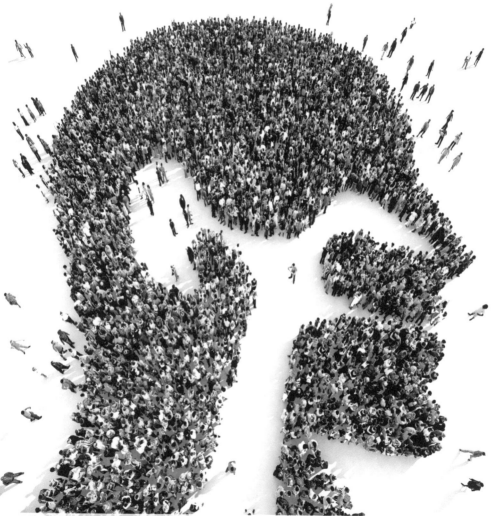

STEVEN OLMOS, DDS
DABCP, DABCDSM, DABDSM, DAIPM, FAAOP, FAACP, FICCMO, FADI, FIAO

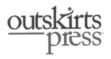

Table of Contents

Foreword

ON A BEAUTIFUL summer day in Scottsdale, Arizona, I began my first lecture in the 2007 conference. I scanned the audience. There was a mix of senior dentistry practitioners and aspiring young dentists who wanted to jump into dental sleep medicine. I couldn't help noticing a man sitting on the left side of the room who looked sophisticated, astute and paid undivided attention to every word I said. As the day went by, I felt how positively he influenced the delivery of my lectures. There was a harmony established. I delivered my best lectures that day. Later in the evening social, I was introduced to him. I knew I had found my match in dental sleep medicine. Dr. Steven Olmos could be a perfect partner in my mission to spread the gospel of sleep.

Indeed, obstructive sleep apnea is an airway problem that adversely affects normal sleep in millions of people around the world. Most of them are left undiagnosed. While lots of work must be done to screen at-risk population, we must treat diagnosed cases with precision and consideration of the airway abnormalities. Sleep apnea causes and worsens medical and mental health conditions including cardiovascular, neuro- cognitive and metabolic complications. It is a significant public health hazard. Annual cost of treating on these conditions exceeds billions of dollars. In addition, it significantly impairs human quality-of-life.

Dr. Steven Olmos is an internationally recognized pioneer in the field of dental sleep medicine. He is the founder of the TMJ & Sleep Therapy Centre International and its over 60 branches in seven countries. He is board-certified in Craniofacial pain and Dental Sleep Medicine. His patented protocols combine both the medical and the dental components of the science of sleep medicine. He served as the president of the American Academy of Craniofacial Pain and Sleep. He has won many accolades, honors and awards. But more importantly, he is a student of sleep science who continuously strives for learning and finding a way to pass his knowledge on to the patients around the world.

Author Dr. Steven Olmos proposes a well-tested solution for the health care crisis that has multiple dimensions. He emphasizes the screening of at-risk population and establishes the relationship between headache, jaw locking, daytime sleepiness and poor nocturnal sleep. He describes five key points of the management based on understanding of airway anatomy and evolutionary function of the nose. Mouth breathing is a critical concept that a practitioner must understand. Current treatment options for sleep apnea and airway management are based on pathophysiologic understanding, philosophy of treatment and author's unparalleled experience. He highlights the finer points by three case studies taken from his own previous publications.

This book is easy to read. Key information is provided in a fluent format, with illustrations further simplifying the critical concepts. The content is supported by an extensive bibliography. This is a 'must read' for Dental practitioners and students alike and is a useful adjunct to medical sleep specialists like myself who work with human airway and obstructive sleep apnea. This supplants airway management in any textbook of sleep medicine.

Deepak Shrivastava, MD, FAASM, FCCP, FACP, RPSGT
Professor of Medicine
UC Davis School of Medicine
Director, Sleep Diagnostics Center SJGH

Who would have thought that clear nasal breathing is so important? They didn't teach us that in medical school.

Dr. Steve Olmos has given us an excellent explanation as to why unobstructed breathing and a full night's sleep are so important to our health.

This book is a much-needed resource for all healthcare providers to screen their patients and to look for and treat the underlying source of their injuries. Individuals with chronic pain will find this book invaluable. Chances are your breathing or, more precisely your obstructive breathing, may be contributing to your misery. Dr. Olmos gives important information on simple measures on how to treat obstructive breathing. It may change your life. Finally, if you have a child who has ADHD, who is a chronic bedwetter, or who has other signs of obstructive breathing, this book may help your child avoid a lifetime of health issues.

Over the years, Dr. Steven Olmos has helped countless chronic pain sufferers around the world by his expertise as well as by his sharing of knowledge to other health care professionals. His keen insight and unyielding compassion for learning and teaching shifted my focus in medicine, making me a better physician. I am certain that this book will help healthcare providers focus on their patient's often neglected breathing issues and help the lay reader live a healthier life.

Victor "Rocky" Romano, OP, MD

A Solution for Our Health Crisis

BREATHING IS VERY important; how well we are able to breathe is closely related to the health of our entire body! The medical community is continuously discovering more and more links between our health problems and poor airway management. Common health issues, such as diabetes, heart (cardiovascular) disease, and high blood pressure, have been found to be connected to the health of the airway. Asthma, a condition where swelling makes it difficult to breathe, is well known, but sleep breathing disorders such as obstructive sleep apnea (OSA) and central sleep apnea (CSA), where breathing becomes difficult or stops during sleep, are not as well known, though they are quite prevalent [1].

Unfortunately, sleep breathing disorders are often not diagnosed by doctors or treated, even though they can be serious and life-threatening [2–4]. Sleep apnea in particular is responsible for more sickness and death than any other sleep disorder. Even though it is found in nearly 11% of the population (about 29.4 million people), only about 20%—a fifth—of these people are diagnosed and treated, leaving 23.5 million people without treatment [5, 6].

There are several reasons why there are such a large number of underdiagnosed and untreated cases of diseases related to breathing, including:

1) a lack of awareness of what signs to look for;
2) a lack of understanding as to how serious these diseases can be; and
3) a healthcare system that is not designed to deal with long-term (chronic) diseases that do not have a "cure."

This means that millions of people continue to suffer from asthma, blocked noses, and pain in the face and jaw despite billions of dollars of healthcare spending. Their airway—the path that air takes through the mouth, nose, sinuses, trachea, and lungs—is not taken care of [4].

In response to this problem, the American Dental Association now requires undergraduate education in sleep breathing, and many schools now offer courses that cover the screening and treatment of sleep breathing disorders. This also helps dental professionals treat their patients without making their conditions worse.

This book will discuss the healthcare problems that can arise from ignoring the airway's effect on the body, and will teach you about airway management—how to take care of the whole airway. It will discuss several techniques that should help patients (and you) breathe easier.

CHAPTER 1

Obstructive Sleep Apnea – What Is It?

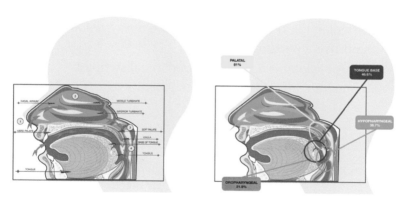

Figure 1 shows the anatomy of the airway. **Figure 2** shows the percentage of OSA-related obstructions for different parts of the airway. *Adapted from: Olmos S. CBCT in the evaluation of airway minimizing orthodontic relapse. Orthodontic Prac. 2015.*

OBSTRUCTIVE SLEEP APNEA (also known as OSA) happens because the airway is blocked or narrowed by something during sleep. It can involve loud snoring and short periods of time where breathing stops. The person begins breathing again within seconds, but it disrupts their sleep and they may wake up several times during the night because of a lack of oxygen. This disrupted pattern of sleep leads to tired brains and bodies, which means more accidents and injuries, poor problem-solving skills, and lowered productivity at work. Lack of sleep is also linked to high blood pressure, heart problems, stroke, and diabetes [7–12]. If these breathing problems continue for a long time, they can cause brain damage in both children and adults [13, 14]. Some individuals with obstructive sleep apnea may also end up being affected by mood issues that hurt other people in their lives [4], and they may abuse tobacco, alcohol, and pills to make up for the lack of deep sleep.

Airway management—through changes in head position, use of supports for the nose and throat, breathing exercises, and other techniques—can help reduce the symptoms of OSA and improve a person's health.

Table 1 contains a summary of clinical symptoms and the sleep breathing disorders they are typically associated with.

Clinical findings that may indicate a risk for sleep-breathing disorders	
Clinical Observation	Potential Relationship
Tongue	
Coated	Risk for gastroesophageal reflux disease from mouth breathing
Enlarged	Increased tongue activity, possible OSA
Scalloping at lateral borders (crenations)	Increased risk for sleep apnea
Obstructs view of oropharynx	Mallampati score of I and II: lower risk for OSA; Mallampati score of III and IV: increased risk for OSA
Teeth and periodontal structure	
Gingival inflammation	Mouth breather; poor oral hygiene
Gingival bleeding when probed	At risk for periodontal disease
Dry mouth (xerostomia)	Mouth breather; may be medication related
Gingival recession	May be at risk for clenching

Tooth wear	May have sleep bruxism
Abfraction (cervical abrasion/wear)	Increased parafunction/clenching
Airway	
Long sloping soft palate	At risk for OSA
Enlarged/swollen/elongated uvula	At risk for OSA/snoring
Extraoral	
Chapped lips for cracking at the corners of the mouth	Inability to nose breathe
Poor lip seal; difficulty maintaining a lip seal	Chronic mouth breather
Mandibular retrognathia	Risk for OSA/snoring
Long face (doliocephalic)	Chronic mouth breathing habit
Enlarged masseter muscle	Clenching/sleep bruxism
Nose/nasal airway	
Small nostrils (nares)	Difficulty nose breathing
Alar rim collapse with forced inspiration	At risk for OSA/sleep-breathing disorder
Posture of the head/neck	
Forward head posture	Airway compromise and restriction
Loss of lordotic curve	Chronic mouth breather
Posterior rotation of the head	Tendency to mouth breathe

Adapted from: Bailey DR. Dentistry's Role in Sleep Medicine (Vol. 5, No. 1). 2010.

There are many factors that may contribute to OSA, and they often work together. Such factors include:

1) People naturally breathe less during sleep.
2) The muscles in the person's throat may have become too weak to hold the airway open while they sleep.
3) The person has enlarged tonsils (an organ at the back of the throat), a naturally small airway, or increased fat deposits near the mouth and "back" of the throat [7].
4) The nose may be blocked by a foreign object, by some part of the nose structure, or by mucus. Infection by bacteria may be a problem as well.

Having a neck circumference (easily measured with a tailors ruler) greater than 17 inches for men and 16 inches for women, and/or having a family history of sleep breathing problems greatly increases the risk of OSA. As we age, sleep breathing problems increase as the tonus of the throat muscles weakens and collapse more frequently and/or completely.

Dentists (and other professionals such as dental hygienists) may be especially valuable for identifying people at risk of breathing problems since they have the opportunity to check on the airways of dental patients at every visit [15, 16]. They can also easily evaluate cases of face or jaw pain, headaches, migraines, and jaw misalignment—all of which might be signs of an airway problem (e.g., SBD) [17, 18, 19]. A lot of these symptoms can be traced back to the grinding of teeth during sleep. Teeth grinding (also known as "sleep bruxism") occurs when there are breathing problems during sleep. It moves the structures of the face around and keeps the airway open. However, this also irritates the muscles in the face and the joints in the jaw, causing pain and stiffness in the face and head [20, 21].

Along with teeth grinding, sleep breathing disorders lead to mouth breathing. This is a reaction to rising carbon dioxide levels (CO_2) in the bloodstream. CO_2 is the endpoint of metabolic activity and is necessary for the release of oxygen from hemoglobin. This is termed the Bohr effect. Breathing through the mouth is the body's attempt to open the airway when the nose is blocked.[22]. Mouth breathing is not good at any time, especially sleep. When mouth breathing you lose CO_2. If enough CO_2 is lost then the body cannot release oxygen from the hemoglobin; it leads to loud sounds such as snoring, increases the risk of infections, and the abnormal mouth breathing alters the way that the skull grows over time, and can lead to changes in the jaw and teeth—such as an open bite [23, 24]. Therefore, if there is mouth breathing and a nose blockage is suspected as the cause, airway management should be started as early as childhood for the best effect on the mouth, skull, and jaw.

Obstructive sleep apnea causes many serious health problems and should be checked and addressed as soon as possible. Dentists and other medical professionals dealing with the mouth, face, teeth, and jaw can catch sleep breathing disorders early on. However, less than half of all dentists can identify the common signs and symptoms of airway disorders, and research shows that while there are high numbers of dental patients (almost one in every three) who might have obstructive sleep apnea, most are not being diagnosed at all [15].

Current Health and Healthcare Statistics

As of 2017, about one out of four Americans had an airway disorder of some sort [33, 36]. Another one in four Americans may develop obstructive sleep apnea in the future. Rising rates of obesity in the United States may increase this number to one in every two [5]. As of 2016, one in three American children and adolescents were deemed as being overweight or obese, reflecting a tripling in obesity rates in children between 1971 and 2011 [25]. Also on the rise are food allergies and allergic reactions to pollen, mold, dust, animals, and other particles. Allergy-related conditions affect millions of Americans each year and can be linked to several problems affecting the airway (such as asthma, sinus infections, and hay fever) [26]. Allergy-related conditions also increase the risk of obstructive sleep apnea.

According to the Centers for Disease Control and Prevention (CDC) and the National Institute of Health (NIH), over 17 million Americans have asthma, 19.1 million received a hay fever diagnosis in 2014, and almost 12% of the U.S. adult population suffers from regular sinus infections [27–30]. The number of people with obstructive sleep apnea will continue to rise with increasing obesity [4], and as climate change leads to warmer seasons and greater pollen production (up to 13–27 days longer for some plants!) [31], related health problems will increase.

Studies also show that there is a clear connection between sleep apnea and pain. This is a significant finding in view of how many people experience chronic pain. In 2014, one in six adults visited the dentist for facial pain, including pain in the jaw and teeth. Women and individuals over 45, in particular, have the most facial pain of any other group [32]. In a 2011 study, at least half of the adults in the U.S. (in 2011) said that they had some form of chronic pain, including pain in the face or teeth. Dealing with this pain, often through the use of painkillers, costs an average of $32 billion annually [32]. Younger people also suffer from chronic pain. Approximately 82% of adolescents report experiencing painful headaches before turning 15 [33–35]. Children who experience chronic tension headaches are more than 15 times more likely to have a sleep breathing disorder, and children with migraines are 8.25 times more likely to do so [36]. Joint pain is also involved, with one in six children and adolescents having a painful jaw problem [37].

People with symptoms of obstructive sleep apnea have been shown to have a 73% higher risk of developing jaw problems such as temporomandibular disease (TMD) [38, 39]. Airway problems in general, such as a narrow or obstructed airway, nasal obstruction or congestion, or mouth breathing during sleep, are linked to a number of painful symptoms, such as: persistent headaches (e.g., migraines, tension headaches), jaw joint inflammation, facial or jaw pain, and tooth damage due to teeth grinding. Medical professionals think that this happens because mouth breathing changes the structure of the jaw and mouth, which causes pain and leads to further problems.

A 2016 study published in the *American Journal of Dentistry* was the first to show that health problems such as headaches and jaw locking are connected to sleepiness in the daytime and poor sleep during the night [40]. Despite this evidence, most patients who seek relief for face or jaw pain do not also have their sleep problems treated.

The incidence of airway-related disorders, including pain, is increasing in the U.S. and throughout the world [41]. Healthcare costs are also going up. According to a 2016 report by the *Journal of the American Medical Association*, people with diabetes spend about $101.4 billion each year, including money spent on medication and emergency care [42]. For people with high blood pressure, it is $83.9 billion per year [42]. These diseases may be linked to airway health. People with chronic pain typically spend about $7,726 more per year on healthcare than an individual with no pain [43], to a total amount of approximately $635 billion in 2012 [43]. In addition, Americans consume 80% of the painkillers that are produced worldwide, and this includes strong—and dangerous—prescription pain medications such as opioids (e.g., Percocet or Vicodin) [44]. The nonmedical use of painkillers (e.g., opioids) costs the U.S. at least $53.4 billion yearly [45].

Undiagnosed obstructive sleep apnea also costs a lot, according to the American Academy of Sleep Medicine [4]. The costs of diagnosis, testing, and follow-up for individuals with obstructive sleep apnea in the United States was $12.4 billion in 2015, while the costs of treating conditions linked to airway problems (e.g., diabetes, TMD, heart disease) and mental health issues for those with undiagnosed OSA was $30 billion. Motor vehicle accidents caused by sleepiness and fatigue resulted in costs of about $26.2 billion in 2015, while workplace accidents and lost productivity resulted in $93.4 billion in financial losses that same year. Treatment, by comparison, saves money. Nonsurgical treatments such as CPAP and oral appliances cost only $6.2 billion, and sleep apnea surgery treatments about $5.4 billion.

Overall, the total healthcare cost in the U.S. in 2015 for people with undiagnosed OSA was $149.6 billion [4]. That's a lot of money being spent on the symptoms of a disease. So why isn't that money being spent on diagnosing and treating the sleep breathing disorder itself, saving money in the long run? The answer to this question lies in the way the healthcare system is structured—and how it focuses on symptoms rather than on the disease as a whole.

What Is the Real Problem?

Because they are often hidden and vary from person to person, finding and taking care of the root causes of illness takes a lot of time and effort—for both patient and doctor. Symptoms are easier—they are visible, and usually what people complain about. They are usually easier to treat, too. That is why the American healthcare system often focuses on the symptoms; it relieves the pain, stops the infections, sets the injuries, and reduces the noise. All this while, it ignores the cause of those symptoms. Doctors frequently don't take a closer look at underlying airway problems, even though treating those problems would help the patient. This isn't the doctor's fault—it's just how they are trained.

A 2015 study revealed that in the dental profession, education typically focuses on diagnosing and managing pain coming from the teeth, gums, and elsewhere in the mouth and face. This includes pain from facial nerves, infections, or jaw problems resulting from mouth breathing [21, 22]. Other types of dental and facial pain, such as pain in the joints and muscles of the jaw, are usually not included [46]. Since they are not looking for the source of the pain—the jaw—they miss the connection between jaw pain, obstructive sleep apnea, and teeth grinding [20, 38, 39]. Instead, they may begin treatment for one or more of the symptoms.

Typical treatments include anticonvulsant medications for blocking pain signals, membrane stabilizing drugs to soothe irritated nerves, and muscle relaxants to relieve tension. These medications may make the patient "feel better" for a time; however, eventually, the patient's body gets used to these medications and they stop being effective. This is called tolerance, and this means that the dose of medication will have to be increased in order to have the same effect. Once the dose reaches a maximum safe amount, then other medications might be added. And so it goes on—the symptoms persist, are treated with increasing amounts of medication, and the underlying cause of the pain is left untreated, causing more problems. It's a broken system.

But it isn't just the doctors that are at fault. Patients with a sleep breathing disorder often ignore their symptoms. In the spirit of "toughing it out," they only go to their primary care physicians when their symptoms become unbearable. Their focus is also the symptoms—they want them to go away. Some patients will attempt to self-medicate, staving off their fatigue and stress with alcohol, tobacco, energy drinks, or energy pills, and using sleeping pills to try to sleep better [47]. Use of these substances leads to other health problems down the road, and may make the underlying issue—the sleep breathing disorder—worse. Smoking, in particular, is known to increase the risk and the intensity of sleep breathing disorders [48], and alcohol may do so as well [49]. Self-medication comes at the cost of learning how to properly manage their airway, and preventing the problem in the first place.

A lack of education on sleep disorders affects both physicians and patients, leading to misdiagnoses as well as prescriptions for unnecessary and potentially harmful sleep medications [50]. Many healthcare providers simply do not recognize the symptoms of breathing conditions, link other common diseases or sleep behaviors to sleep quality, or don't consider sleep breathing disorders to be important at all! This leaves approximately 23.5 million people without the correct diagnosis, and without treatment [5, 6].

On the other hand, even for those who have been diagnosed with a sleep breathing disorder, treatment options are limited. A continuous positive airway pressure (CPAP) device, a machine that pumps air into their nose to help with breathing, is the most commonly used treatment. Oral orthotics and surgery are also available, as is therapy and lifestyle changes [4]. Proper body positioning during sleep or weight loss regimens can also be used; however, these treatments vary in effectiveness and mainly treat the symptoms, not the deeper problems that may be causing the airway condition in the first place.

The situation regarding sleep breathing disorders reflects a failure of the healthcare system as a whole. Dealing with it requires a complete overhaul of how medicine as a profession is taught, and how doctors are expected to deal with their patients. Change will be difficult ... but not impossible.

What Is the Solution?

Solving the problem of underdiagnosed sleep breathing disorders could be as simple as asking people "can you get to sleep?" "can you stay asleep" and "do you wake rested?" This draws out answers that can help a doctor see if there is a sleep disorder, and signals to the patients that they should pay attention to how well they are sleeping. This is a part of "screening"—a process that tries to identify patients with problems before these problems get out of hand.

It is best to do screening as early as possible, even in infancy, since jaw joint and sleep breathing problems can change the bone structure and sleep behaviors of children as they grow. When caught early in childhood or adolescence, it is often possible to cure their airway problem through a medical or dental intervention. When diagnosed during adulthood, however, these types of health issues can usually only be managed, not fixed [25]. The American Academy of Pediatrics recommends that all children and teenagers should be screened for snoring and asthma. If there are problems, the academy also recommends that the children be tested for a sleep disorder, usually through a sleep study (polysomnography) [47, 51].

Because of the connection between chronic pain and breathing, dentists can become a first line of defense against long-term problems by screening for airway difficulties that may be linked to their patients' discomfort. Dr. Christian Guilleminault (pioneer of sleep medicine) emphasized the important role that the field of orthodontics plays in the diagnosis and treatment of breathing disorders. "One can see," he said in his coauthored editorial "Orthodontics and Sleep Disordered Breathing," "that the role of dentists and orthodontists has become very important and will continue to grow even further in the years to come" [52].

However, there needs to be a better understanding of what causes breathing problems, and what to look for when a patient comes in to the doctor. When presented with face or jaw pain, medical professionals need to be trained to look for an airway problem as a potential underlying cause. They should check the airway after certain incidents that could cause problems, or make existing problems worse; for example, neck and face traumas [53].

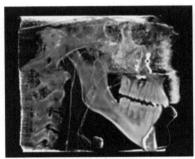 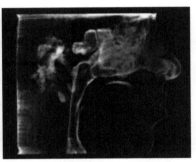

Figure 3 and Figure 4. *Adapted from: Olmos S. CBCT in the evaluation of airway minimizing orthodontic relapse. Orthodontic Prac. 2015.*

Treatment also needs to be improved. Because a healthy airway could reduce the risks of many different health ailments, such as diabetes and high blood pressure, the focus should be on maintaining a healthy airway. Clinical evidence supports this, showing that proper treatment for obstructed breathing disorders lowers the risk of high blood pressure and diabetes [54, 55].

Treating an airway disorder involves five key points: inflammation control, jaw joint correction, taking care of irritated muscles in the face, keeping the airway free of obstructions (such as swelling), and having a balanced diet that reduces inflammation [18]. Treatment reduces sleep disturbances, which also reduces the risk of heart disease [57], sugar (glucose) intolerance, and insulin resistance (which can lead to the development of diabetes) [58], making treatment an even more beneficial option.

Finally, there needs to be more awareness of how important airway management is to overall health—and the consequences of not catching and treating problems. Again, this is not just the responsibility of medical professionals—changes need to be made in how patients address sleep disorders. It is important that individuals do not try to "tough out" their loud snoring or persistent sleepiness. Society at large needs to consider these things as serious health problems, not a consequence of poor lifestyle habits or "laziness."

Better screening, treatment, knowledge, and awareness of airway problems will lead to better health overall. In the following chapters, we will go into more depth about how the airway works and what treatments are currently available for use. However, in the meantime, every medical or dental visit is an opportunity to conduct airway disorder screening—and a chance to catch a breathing disorder before it becomes a problem.

CHAPTER 2

Screening for Obstructive Sleep Apnea

OBSTRUCTIVE SLEEP APNEA is usually diagnosed through a sleep study called a polysomnography. Polysomnography, or PSG, is usually done at a sleep center, a hospital, or at home through a sleep apnea test. Multiple appointments and an overnight sleep test in a special facility may be needed to detect the problem. An at-home sleep apnea test is less expensive and more convenient than one that is performed at a sleep center, but it cannot track periods of sleep and wakefulness, and might miss some cases of sleep apnea. It may also miss breathing problems where the person wakes up periodically, but may not actually stop breathing. The stress that this causes, called an "arousal," can be detected at a sleep center.

To complicate matters, health insurance coverage for both types of tests varies by payer, geographic region, and availability [4]. However, when sleep breathing disorders are caught and treated through airway management early on, healthcare costs and out-of-pocket spending are reduced. For example, a survey found that, when treated, about 3% of the patients who had obstructive sleep apnea and high blood pressure were able to stop taking their medication, while 17% were able to take a lower dose. For those who had diabetes, receiving treatment for a breathing disorder dramatically reduced their average number of hospital visits from 2.8 to 1.5. When they improved their airway management, they improved their overall health and reduced their overall healthcare costs—making airway management a cost-effective option, even with uncertain insurance.

What Is the Function of the Nose?

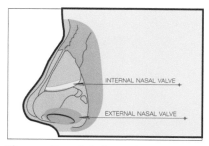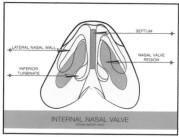

Figures 5 and 6 show the anatomy of the unobstructed nose.
Adapted from: Olmos S. CBCT in the evaluation of airway minimizing orthodontic relapse. Orthodontic Prac. 2015.

The nose is an organ for breathing and smelling. Although the mouth is also connected to the airway, it is better to breathe through the nose because air is filtered, moistened, and warmed as it is drawn through the nose. Warm, moist air prevents the delicate tissue of the airway from becoming damaged. Mucus and tiny hairs on the inside of the nose catch dust, bacteria, viruses, and pollen before they can get inside.

Additionally, nasal breathing draws nitric oxide (NO) from the sinuses allowing it to mix with incoming air. Nitric oxide kills funguses, bacteria, and viruses that would make us sick, and also helps blood vessels expand. This improves blood flow in the airway and lets more oxygen pass into the body—about 10 to 15% more than mouth-breathing can provide [59]. Nitric oxide also causes tiny hairs in the nose to move. They "beat" back foreign particles, forcing them out of the nose and preventing infection [23].

Even though it is best to breathe through the nose, because it is narrow it can become blocked for many different reasons. Narrow or collapsed nostrils might restrict airflow [59]. The nose could be dislocated, or the separating wall (also known as the septum) between the nostrils might be shifted to one side or the other (a deviated septum), narrowing the airway. There could even be a noncancerous growth inside the nostril. Typically, these conditions are treated through surgery [60].

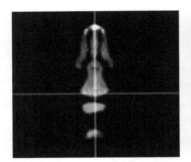 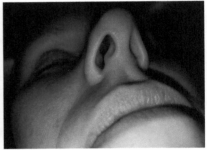

Figure 7 shows the computed tomography image of the obstructed airway for the patient shown on the right **Figure 8** shows nasal valve obstruction
Adapted from: Olmos S. CBCT in the evaluation of airway minimizing orthodontic relapse. Orthodontic Prac. 2015.

Another type of blockage comes from irritation and inflammation in the nasal passage, leading to a high amount of mucus in the nose. This is known as congestion [61]. Often caused by allergies, this usually involves a "runny" or "stuffy" nose, sinus pain, and a buildup of mucus that can make it difficult to breathe. Congestion will be covered in greater detail in the next chapter.

Since the nose is the natural way to breathe, and a major way that the body protects itself from being invaded by harmful toxins, bacteria, and viruses, it is important to deal with any blockages as soon as possible. This is especially important for children; nose obstruction or congestion in infants can prevent them from eating and lead to life-threatening breathing problems. Nasal blockages can even cause hearing and speech problems because of their effect on the eustachian tubes—a set of organs that connect the nose to the throat and the middle ear [62]. A blocked or inflamed nasal passage causes fluids to build up in the inner ear, putting pressure on these tubes and resulting in pain and hearing loss. If left untreated, nose blockages or other abnormalities can affect head posture, body posture, chronic facial pain, sleep breathing, the formation of facial structures, and the risk of getting cavities in the teeth, among other things.

Because of its effect on the health of the entire body, the nose should be well cared for.

Mouth Breathing – Why It Happens and What It Does to the Airway

The mouth, though it is a larger opening than the nose, is not the best way to breathe; it doesn't have filter hairs, mucus, or nitric oxide. This means that infections are more likely with mouth breathing, and the body doesn't take in as much oxygen. Other risks come from breathing through the mouth as well, such as choking—which can be life threatening—and dehydration of the airway tissues, which can lead to damage and irritation of the throat and lungs.

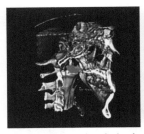 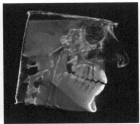 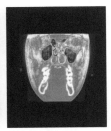

Figure 9 on the left shows a narrow throat that is obstructing the airway. **Figure 10** in the middle shows an i-CAT image that is used to identify airway obstructions. **Figure 11** on the right shows total nasal obstruction due to swollen nasal tissue.
Adapted from: Olmos S. CBCT in the evaluation of airway minimizing orthodontic relapse. Orthodontic Prac. 2015.

Of course, sometimes it is necessary to breathe through the mouth, such as when the nose is blocked. This is because the body can only survive for a few minutes without oxygen. While asleep, the brain keeps track of breathing. If it detects that there is a problem with breathing, it makes muscles in the face contract, leading to teeth grinding or clenching during sleep. This helps to keep air moving through the airway. If these movements are not enough, the mouth is opened. Though this is important to survival, the movements of the muscles also damage them, as well as the nerves in the face [18, 22]. They react to this damage by producing free radicals (a toxic waste product that is involved in cancers and age-related diseases), neurotransmitters (chemicals that allow neurons to "talk" to each other), and the release of white blood cells (immune system cells that help to fight infection) [63]. This causes further damage to the tissues of the airway and more pain.

Pain from jaw clenching during sleep includes tension headaches and pain in the base of the skull [64]. Jaw joint, sinus, or dental problems can also cause headaches. The jaw joints are especially important; because they connect the jaw to the skull, they are involved with such commonplace actions as talking, chewing, and breathing through the mouth. Muscles in the jaw region, the cheeks, the top of the head, and at the sides are involved with the movement of the jaw— so if a jaw joint problem (such as temporomandibular disease) is causing abnormal jaw movement, or if a blockage in the nose causes the mouth to remain open for longer periods than normal, then muscles all over the head are affected. The pain resulting from these strained and damaged muscles can affect the ears, teeth, neck, and shoulders.

Mouth breathing also dries out the mouth. Saliva washes away excess food, kills bacteria, and washes away dead bacteria. This protects the mouth from infection. Breathing through the mouth leads to low amounts of saliva—and an increased risk for cavities, tooth decay, bad breath, and gum disease [65]. A dry mouth also means that the air reaching the throat and lungs is not moist enough. This dry air, combined with the higher levels of airborne particles that come from mouth breathing, may also cause adenoids and tonsils to swell [7]. Tonsils and adenoids help regulate the immune system, working together with nose hairs and mucus to stop toxins and harmful bacteria from entering your body. Unfortunately, when they become swollen, they cannot do their job, and instead reduce or block the flow of air through the nose—leading to or worsening mouth breathing [7].

Research also indicates that mouth breathing can affect the entire spine and result in abnormal back, abdominal, and pelvic posture [66]. Poor posture can lead to muscle tension, pain, and slouching. This makes the early diagnosis and treatment of mouth breathing very important. Usually, mouth breathing is diagnosed by checking for teeth grinding or snoring. However, night guards—a common treatment to prevent teeth grinding and snoring—can make sleep breathing disorders worse [67].

Therefore, treatments that target the blockage that is causing mouth breathing are important, and can lead to better long-term health.

Relationship between the Nose, Dental Problems, and Facial Malformation

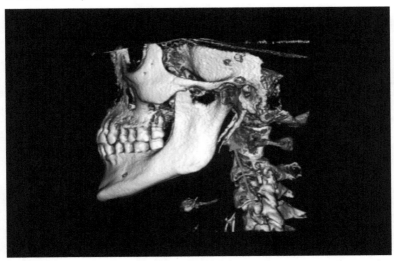

Figure 12 shows elongated styloid processes (bones in the neck), which indicates long-standing motor activity of the jaw (e.g., chronic mouth breathing) to maintain an open airway.

Adapted from: Olmos S. CBCT in the evaluation of airway minimizing orthodontic relapse. Orthodontic Prac. 2015.

One of the posture changes that breathing and jaw problems cause is forward head posture (FHP), where the head is held forward and rotated from the torso. For every inch that the head is placed in front of the shoulders, an extra 10 pounds of weight is placed on the neck and spine. This leads to pain in the neck and lower back, abnormal curvature of the neck, and slumped shoulders [68, 69]. The additional weight may also pinch nerves and cause problems with bone growth, such as osteoarthritis [70].

Facial structure also depends on the state of the nose. This is because, when you breathe through your nose, the tongue normally rests against the roof of the mouth, and the cheeks press inward. This constant, gentle pressure causes the bones of the mouth to grow into a "U-shaped" upper arch. However, during mouth breathing, the tongue is no longer pressed against the roof of your mouth. Instead of the proper "U shape," a "V-shaped arch" may develop. "V-shaped arches" can cause the teeth in the mouth to become crowded, lead to an overbite, and can cause problems with swallowing [24].

Figure 14 shows scalloping of the tongue, which refers to the appearance of indentations on the sides of the tongue due to it being consistently pressed against the teeth.

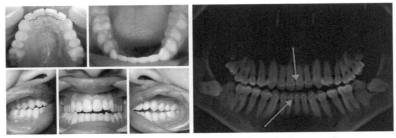

Figure 13 shows an open bite that developed due to the tongue pushing the teeth forward in order to maintain an open airway.
Adapted from: Olmos S. CBCT in the evaluation of airway minimizing orthodontic relapse. Orthodontic Prac. 2015.

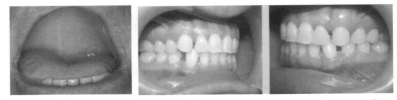

Figure 14 on the left shows the tongue retracting as the mouth is opened and scalloping of the tongue, which is 70% predictive of OSA. **Figure 15** on the right shows gaps between the teeth that developed due to the tongue pushing against the front teeth to maintain an open airway.
Adapted from: Olmos S. CBCT in the evaluation of airway minimizing orthodontic relapse. Orthodontic Prac. 2015.

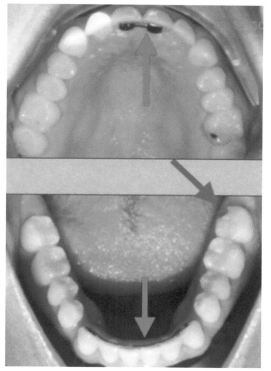

Figure 16. Forward tooth movement due to obstruction indicated by green arrows and a fractured molar indicated by a purple arrow due to bruxism (teeth clenching and grinding).
Adapted from: Olmos S. CBCT in the evaluation of airway minimizing orthodontic relapse. Orthodontic Prac. 2015.

Normally, during swallowing, the tongue should stay firmly pressed against the top of the mouth, and with the teeth in contact. This supports the muscles involved in swallowing and allows it to proceed smoothly. With mouth breathing, the tongue remains at the bottom of the mouth and may even begin to press against the lower front teeth. This changes the position of the lower jaw and the lower teeth, causing them to shift forward. That may result in the front teeth not touching (anterior open bite).

Keeping the mouth open for a long period of time also causes muscle fatigue as in mouth breathing. This is abnormal, as the mouth should be closed when proper nasal breathing is utilized. Chronic mouth breathing means that any activity using those muscles will result in pain and limited movement. Examples would be speaking, eating, or having dental work. It can also result in a dislocation of the jaw joints preventing opening or having the jaw locked open and unable to close without manipulation. The mechanism is that this shifts the jaw backward, causing the jaw joint to rub against the bone socket it is in, resulting in a clicking or popping noise. This is easily heard and felt, and is one of the main symptoms of temporomandibular disease [71]. This places pressure on nerves that connect the ear to the brain, and may result in ear itching, pain, and other ear pathology like ear congestion or ear ringing (tinnitus) [72].

The teeth are also influenced by infections in the nose via a different route. The roots of the upper teeth are close to the sinuses, and sinus infections may spread to the gums and teeth. This works both ways: cavities, impacted teeth, or abscesses (an infection at a tooth's root) can also cause sinus infections [73]. An infection of the gums or gum disease can become especially dangerous because bacteria can travel from the gums into the bloodstream, where they can spread throughout the body and cause further disease.

Sleep Breathing Disorders and Sleep Disturbances

The normal sleep cycle lasts for 90 minutes so in a normal sleep a person should have 4-5 sleep cycles. Optimum sleep for an adult is 7 hours. Normal sleep consists of two parts: non-REM sleep and REM sleep. REM refers to rapid eye movement, which can be seen during this stage of sleep. Dreaming and problem solving also take place during REM sleep. REM sleep accounts for about 20 to 25% of normal sleep, while non-REM sleep occurs for the remainder and encourages healing and rest. While both parts of sleep are important, it is REM sleep that promotes attention and learning while people are awake [74].

It is also REM sleep that is disturbed by sleep breathing disorders. This leads to headaches, fatigue, problems with mood, and pain. The sleep conditions caused by sleep breathing disorders include [75]:

- Dyssomnia – Excessive daytime sleepiness that can increase the risks of accidents, and cause issues with problem solving and productivity at work or school.
- Insomnia – Poor sleep quality or the absence of normal sleep cycles.
- Parasomnia – Unusual behavior during sleep, including sleepwalking, sleep aggression, and sleep paralysis.
- Movement Disorder – Unusual and unconscious movements, such as restless leg syndrome and teeth grinding.

The pain that comes with sleep breathing disorders (such as jaw, neck, and back pain) can also cause problems more directly. Constant pain causes a condition called "central sensitization," where a person becomes more sensitive to pain. Basically, pain leads to more pain. This releases cortisol, a stress hormone that increases heart rate and blood volume, and speeds up metabolism. Metabolism changes make people more vulnerable to conditions such as diabetes [47, 51] and can cause frequent headaches and insomnia [76]. This relationship between sleep problems and pain has been researched for a long time [77–79]. Cluster headaches in particular are known to awaken individuals from their sleep around the same time every night. These particular headaches are very painful and are caused by low levels of oxygen in the blood (oxygen is often used to treat these headaches) [74]. The combination of low oxygen and pain forces people to wake up.

With obstructive sleep apnea, people may stop breathing for at least 10 seconds. A person suffering from this disorder will wake up repeatedly during the night, either completely or partially, to breathe. This disturbs their sleep and leads to fatigue and sleepiness while awake. It often results in irregular snoring, choking, or gasping as well. This lack of sleep can affect the brain, causing personality changes, memory problems, and irritability. It can also cause morning headaches and acid reflux. If it is left untreated, this will worsen over time. Men aged 40 to 60 are most at risk for OSA, but a family history of breathing problems, obesity, high blood pressure, tobacco, alcohol, or sedative use, asthma and allergies, hormone changes from menopause, crowded teeth, and teeth grinding are also risk factors [74].

The Ins and Outs of Congestion

Congestion—a "stuffed" or "runny" nose that is difficult to breathe through—is caused by mucus buildup or inflammation. Mucus in the nose is normal; it lines the mouth, throat, nose, and lungs and serves several purposes:

- It protects the lining of the airways from becoming dry.

- It traps allergens (such as dust or pollen) and bacteria, preventing them from entering the body and causing sickness.
- It destroys bacteria and viruses with antibodies and enzymes [80].

Mucus protects the body. However, when a person gets sick or is exposed to large amounts of allergens, mucus begins to work against them. The immune system reacts to the threat by producing more mucus than normal, clogging the nose and blocking the airway. This leads to a runny nose, itching, sneezing, and stuffiness. An infection in the nasal passage can also cause thick mucus that is usually yellow and becomes green in color as the infection gets worse [80]. This can drip down the throat and spread the infection.

Inflammation—the swelling of tissue and blood vessels in the nasal passage—also causes congestion. Any type of damage to the nasal passages activates the immune system, which releases special hormones called histamines [80]. Histamines do three very important things:

1) They signal the body to expand the blood vessels at the irritated area—in this case, the nose. This way, more blood can reach that area.
2) The walls of these blood vessels also expand so that fluid, immune system cells, and particles important to healing can gather in the area, where they are needed.
3) Third, histamines signal the body to make special types of white blood cells called neutrophils and macrophages which destroy and "eat" harmful substances, clearing them from the body.

The short-term inflammation that results from the activity of histamines is actually beneficial. However, if inflammation continues for a long time, it can cause serious health problems, and often hints at a deeper issue.

Long-term inflammation can happen if there are harmful substances that can't be destroyed. It can also happen if there are allergens that are setting off the immune system. The immune system overreacts to usually harmless substances, sending too much fluid, too many immune system cells, and too many healing particles to a site. This means that they build up, cause swelling, and may even begin to destroy healthy tissue [80]. This causes pain at the site, and even bleeding.

Dryness of the nose causes inflammation and leads to congestion. One of the main causes of this dryness is allergies. Over the last ten years, the presence of allergies has increased dramatically in infants, children, adolescents, and adults [81]. According to research, this increase is because of air pollution, changes in the environment, processed food, and the increased use of antihistamines, antibiotics, and other medications that weaken the immune system [81–84]. Increased carbon monoxide (CO) from car emissions as well as increased CO_2 levels and warmer temperatures lead to larger numbers of allergens in the air [85]. This makes it harder for the body's natural defenses to filter the air that we breathe, and leaves high levels of these particles in the airway to irritate it. Cooling and heating appliances can also dry out the air, leading to dry sinuses, making allergy symptoms worse, and increasing the risk of sinus or upper respiratory infections [86]. Together, this can cause serious congestion even in people without allergies.

Animal dander is a common household allergen that inflames the airway and causes a buildup of mucus. Many people now own animals such as birds, hamsters, guinea pigs, rabbits, and other exotic pets in addition to cats and dogs, and this has resulted in a higher rate of allergy-related health problems [87]. Some airborne allergens such as cat dander are so tiny that they can travel deep into the airways—even the lungs—where they can trigger asthma-like symptoms. Dander can stay in the air for a long period of time, up to six to nine months after an animal has been removed from the home; therefore, even a clean, animal-free home might still cause problems for a long time [87].

Food allergies to artificial flavors, preservatives, colors, proteins, and chemical ingredients can also lead to inflammation and life-threatening swelling in the tongue, lips, and throat. The use of prescription medication and over-the-counter medicine can also cause allergic reactions, and certain medications can even reduce the body's natural ability to fight off harmful bacteria and viruses [87, 82–84].

CHAPTER 3

Treatments for Obstructive Sleep Apnea

THERE ARE THREE treatment options that are currently available for sleep breathing disorders:

- Continuous positive airway pressure devices (also known as CPAP devices)
- Surgery
- Oral orthotics for use in the mouth

Diet and breathing exercises are also options.

Surgery is generally only recommended when the problem is physical, such as enlarged tonsils or adenoids, unusual nose structures, or swollen throat structures, and is affecting the patient's breathing.

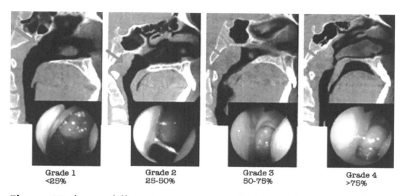

| Grade 1 | Grade 2 | Grade 3 | Grade 4 |
| <25% | 25-50% | 50-75% | >75% |

Figure 17 shows different percentages of airway obstruction due to swollen tonsils or adenoids.
Adapted from: Olmos S. CBCT in the evaluation of airway minimizing orthodontic relapse. Orthodontic Prac. 2015.

The following sections describe the strengths and weaknesses of each of the nonsurgical treatments.

Continuous Positive Airway Pressure (CPAP) Devices

A continuous positive airway pressure (CPAP) device is a ventilator that applies air pressure to keep the airway open via a mask that is placed over the face.

CPAP devices work very well; however, they do come with some side effects, such as rawness and irritation of the throat, congestion of the nose, cuts on the bridge of the nose from the mask, and sleep problems from the noise of the machine. It also puts pressure on the face, which can make some sleep breathing disorders worse. The noise is also disturbing to people sleeping next to the patient, and the device cannot be easily moved. So, even though it is a highly effective method to treat a sleep breathing disorder, doctors should carefully consider what is causing the sleep breathing disorder before they prescribe a CPAP device [88].

Oral Appliance Therapy

Oral appliances are structures that are worn in the mouth to support the jaw joint and hold the airway open. Oral appliances are noninvasive and are usually only worn during the day or night, though sometimes both. Day appliances are usually for the jaw, while night appliances are usually used to treat airway obstructions and sleep breathing problems. Narrow airways, painful muscle contractions in the jaw, and frequent tension headaches are treated by appliances that can be worn during the day and the night [89].

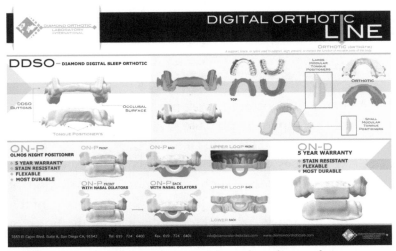

Figure 18. Appliances used to provide oral appliance therapy.

Clinical research involving participants with temporo-mandibular disease shows that when oral appliances are used properly, they give people relief from joint pain, face pain, ear pain, headaches, ringing in the ears, and poor posture for the long term [90, 91]. A person wearing a custom fitted oral appliance should closely follow directives of the dental professional on its use. Success of treatment is dependent on how well the person adheres to the recommended regimen. If a person has never worn a dental appliance then it may take a little time to acclimate. Oral appliances are necessary for healing, protecting against further injury, or used to maintain breathing during sleep, often all of the above. Immediately upon removal a person's bite may be different due to the positioning of the jaw during the time the appliance has been worn. This often can be reversed by opening and closing the mouth a couple of times, or by gently pressing the teeth together for two or three seconds, repeating the movement until the bite returns to normal.

Daytime oral appliances are not recommended for extended periods of use, and may not be appropriate for some breathing disorders (such as a blocked nose) [89].

Pediatric Treatment for OSA

Finding and treating obstructive sleep apnea in children reduces their risk for other diseases. Since adults who have sleep breathing disorders must be treated for life [92, 93], whereas a child who is being treated will significantly reduce the disorders effect later in life, it is especially important to diagnosis this disorder as early as possible.

The reported rates for obstructive sleep apnea in children are 1.2% to 5.7% [95–96], but this may be a low estimate because of the lack of proper screening in children. Snoring is a key symptom of a sleep breathing disorder, and approximately 10% of children snore on a regular basis [97, 98].

In 2012, the American Academy of Pediatrics recommended that all children and adolescents be screened for snoring and that sleep studies be performed if they showed symptoms of a sleep breathing disorder [99].

Other symptoms of sleep breathing disorders in children include teeth grinding, forward head posture, bed-wetting, restless sleep, and ADHD, among others. Bedwetting, in relation to sleep breathing disorders, can be caused by negative pressure on the ribcage from the diaphragm trying to draw air into the body with resistance from an obstruction of the throat (tongue). The pressure causes extra blood to pool in the right atrium. The extra blood results in a false fluid overlaod, triggers Atrial Natriuretic Peptide (ANP) and produces more urine to balance the perceived fluid overload. Children sleep deeply, they sleep through the urge to urinate.

Additional problems associated with sleep breathing disorders in children include [25, 98]:

1) Poor growth hormone production that results in reduced growth and body development,
2) Slowed heart rate and low blood oxygen levels that are linked to high blood pressure or additional heart and lung issues, and
3) Higher risk of obesity due to increased resistance to insulin—the hormone that helps break down sugars in the blood—and increased tiredness that reduces physical activity.

Screening for a sleep breathing disorder should be performed if a child suffers from snoring, unexplained bed-wetting, gasping for air, mood changes, behavioral issues, dramatic weight changes, and facial pain [25].

Certain treatments for obstructive sleep apnea should not be used on children. Certain oral appliances and the headgear used for CPAP devices may prevent the bones of the child's face from growing properly. Similarly, nasal corrective surgery, tongue reduction, and uvulopalatopharyngoplasty (UPPP) surgery (a surgery to correct the uvula) should not be used for children [97]. A useful treatment for children, however, is expanding the upper jaw. It increases the space available for air to travel through the nose, making it easier to breathe.

Clinical research shows that palatal (upper jaw) expansion [92, 100–105]:

- restores proper nasal breathing
- reduces apnea events
- increases the air volume of the nose
- straightens posture
- corrects skeletal deformities that block breathing
- improves conductive hearing loss, fatigue, and bed-wetting

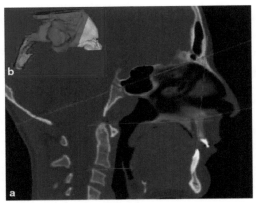

Figure 19. Shows a 2.36% nasal volume increase for each mm of palatal expansion.
Adapted from: Motro M, Schauseil M, Ludwig B, et al. Rapid-maxillary expansion induced rhinological effects: a retrospective multicenter study. Eur Arch Otorhinolaryngol. 2016; 273(3):679–87.

Tips for Managing Congestion

Nasal congestion, inflammation, and irritation that is accompanied by mucus buildup make it hard to breathe through your nose. This can lead to additional problems such as headaches, blocked ears, snoring, and disturbed sleep. Fortunately, there are certain strategies that can help relieve nasal congestion. These are:

- Nasal washes or rinses,
- Certain breathing exercises,
- Eating a healthy diet,
- And treating blockages in the nose.

These will be discussed in detail in this section [60].

Saline Sinus Irrigation

Allergies, hay fever, chronic sinus infections, or asthma can block the nose and cause breathing disorders. Most allergens that trigger these issues are not easily avoided, but there are several natural approaches to airway management that help the body resist allergies. These approaches include: steam inhalation, nasal saline irrigation, and xylitol nasal irrigation.

Steam inhalation thins the mucus, allowing it to drain out of the nose. It also eases swelling in the nasal passage. It is one of the easiest methods to put into action. All you need is a source of steam and the ability to breathe (at least a little bit) through the nose.

Saline sinus irrigation, or nasal rinsing, flushes the nose with saltwater or a saline spray. The rinse can be performed with a squirt or spray bottle, or a device with a nasal spout such as a neti pot, which is a container that uses gravity to pull the water through the nose [106]. As it moves through the nasal passage, the water washes out pollen, dust, and excess mucus [107]. It also helps the nose restore the thin layer of mucus that prevents irritants, allergens, viruses, and bacteria from remaining in the nose and passing into the airway and the bloodstream.

Sinus irrigation also clears out excess or hardened mucus and reduces coughing caused by postnasal drip. It can safely be used by adults and children, and does not cause serious side effects [108–110]. In fact, research shows that using nasal rinses reduces the use of medication and trips to the doctor for allergy problems [108, 111, 112].

Nasal rinses have been in use for hundreds of years as an Ayurvedic medical tradition. In the 1900s, its use expanded to several countries, including the U.S., for the treatment of allergies [113, 114]. Research indicates that physicians often recommend this technique for chronic nasal congestion [106, 113–115], but they do not always suggest it as the first line of defense against allergies. As a result, this approach is not being used to its fullest extent.

There are certain cases where a nasal rinse is not enough, though. For example, a serious sinus or lung infection would require treatment with medication. Additionally, performing sinus irrigation regularly for a long time may lead to dryness and irritation in the nose, which could lead to infection and other problems [110]. However, because of the health benefits it provides, it should still be used when a nasal problem is discovered, and less frequently after the symptoms have stopped, to prevent future flare-ups.

Sinus Irrigation with Xylitol Saline Solution

Xylitol is a form of sugar alcohol that can easily be combined with saline (natural saltwater). This particular mixture moisturizes the nasal passage and also boosts the body's natural antibacterial activity [116]. Xylitol saline sinus irrigation washes out and cleanses the nasal passage more thoroughly than saline sinus irrigation, which simply rinses the nasal passage. More specifically, xylitol solution boosts the thin protective layer of mucus that lines the airway.

This protective mucus contains several proteins, enzymes, and other potent substances that help it fight off infectious agents [29]. These substances are actually a part of the body's natural defense against bacteria, viruses, pollen, and additional environmental irritants that can be inhaled through the mouth or nose.

However, the thin layer of mucus is sensitive to changes in its salt level—changes caused by allergens, bacteria, and viruses.

Xylitol saline solution helps lower the salt concentration, allowing the mucus to better protect the airways [116]. This type of salt-reducing solution has been used for patients with bronchiectasis (lung inflammation and damage) and cystic fibrosis (a devastating inherited lung disease) to reduce coughing and to help clear out excess mucus [117]. Xylitol itself creates a protective layer in the nose that bacteria can't stick to or grow on, reducing the risk of infection further [116, 118]. This means that, while washing out the nose with a saline solution is good, using xylitol is better.

A good over the counter product is Xlear which is comprised of hyperosmotic saline and xylitol. Xlear's formulation of saline is identical to the saline content in human cells. This is optimal for the rehydration of nasal tissues.

Breathing Exercises

In addition to performing sinus irrigation, there are a number of breathing exercises that not only reduce congestion, but also strengthen the respiratory muscles. Several of these techniques are supported by research, and most of the approaches can easily be incorporated into a normal daily routine.

One type of breathing exercise is known as pranayama [119]. This is a breathing exercise from the yoga tradition that involves sitting comfortably in a relaxed, but upright, position and taking several deep breaths through the nose, and then exhaling forcefully and quickly (again through the nose) in short, one-second bursts. This is done 10 times before relaxing into a normal breathing pattern. The breathing exercise can be extended to 20 or 30 exhales, and can be done during a warm shower. This helps to loosen mucus, reduce pressure on the sinuses, and decrease pain in the sinuses and nose.

Breathing in this way also boosts the flow of oxygen into the bloodstream, which feeds the brain, heart, and lungs and improves overall health. It also relieves headaches. A study showed that six weeks of pranayama breathing led to heightened airflow throughout the respiratory system [120]. Another study suggests that this form of breathing can strengthen the lung muscles [121], and makes breathing easier [119]. Research even suggests that this form of exercise reduces stress and anxiety, improves blood circulation and the breakdown of sugars in the body, and can improve the health of patients with cancer [122–126].

Breathing through the nose, meaning inhaling and exhaling through the nose is the only proper way to breathe, both day and night. CO_2 (carbon dioxide) is the driving force for stimulation of breathing. It is necessary in the lungs and in arteries to release oxygen from the red blood cells (hemoglobin). This is called the Bohr effect for the doctor who discovered this effect. Depletion of CO_2 from mouth breathing results in all of the cells in our body starving for oxygen. This lowers the pH of the blood resulting in acidic levels. [128]

Exercises to check to see if you have the proper level would be to see how many seconds it takes after inhaling and exhaling a nasal breath to feel the first desire to breathe. Less than 20 seconds and you have a nasal breathing problem (mouth breathing). People with asthma, and or hyperventilation syndrome can often have as little as 3 to 5 seconds before they need to breathe.

Breathing exercises such as Buteyko can increase the volume of air you breathe and restore proper balance of CO_2

and O2. This is good for us in everyday life and in sports. Patrick McKeown is the author of books on this technique: "The Oxygen Advantage", and "Close Your Mouth".

For people with nasal congestion simply holding your breath for as long as you can after a normal inhalation and exhalation through the nose while swaying will open nasal airway. The person should gently sway from side to side while doing this exercise. This should be repeated five times with a 60 second rest between exercises. Do not use this forceful breath holding technique if you have asthma, hyperventilation syndrome, or anxiety.

Most people who have had nasal surgery still have blocked nasal air flow. This is due to the first point of entry being blocked, the nasal valve. In the past and even now most ENT surgeons ignore the nasal valve. Nasal dilators are necessary for these people. Breathe right, nasal cones and other devices will enhance sleep as well as the exercises. This is true even for the people that use CPAP devices, and or oral appliances for people with obstructive sleep apnea/snoring.[129, 130, 131, 132)

There are new surgeries that are simple recontouring techniques that can be done in the surgeons' office with only local anesthesia. Often taking as little as 15 minutes for people with this problem. You can tell if have a nasal valve problem by using the Cottle's maneuver [133]. This is a simple technique of breathing normally through the nose to establish the usual flow and then placing your thumb and index fingers on the cheek bones and lifting up. If this improves you nasal airflow then you have a nasal valve limitation.

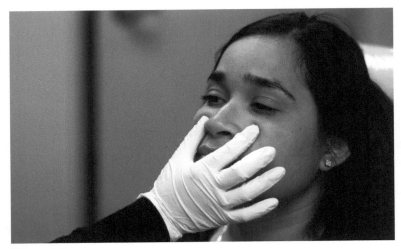

Figure 20

In addition to breathing techniques, a humidifier should be run at night to put moisture in the air. Some humidifiers have a slot for adding menthol oil such as peppermint or eucalyptus. These types of oils also help open the airways.

Additional recommendations to help with airway problems include [87, 107]:

- Regularly changing the air filters in air-conditioning/heating units
- Monitoring pollen counts and avoiding outdoor activities when the pollen count is high
- Showering in the morning and at night to wash pollen and other airborne irritants off of the skin and hair
- Testing for allergens using a skin test, and then avoiding any that cause a reaction
- Removing dust mites and animal dander from surfaces, and wearing a mask while cleaning to reduce irritant exposure

- Washing bedding frequently and vacuuming regularly with a high-efficiency particulate (HEPA) filter, if possible

Nutrition for Breathing

What you eat determines how well you sleep. Current research shows that a diet that is low in fiber but high in saturated fat and processed sugar causes lighter, less restorative sleep, with more frequent awakening and more sleepiness the next day [135]. The less sleep someone has, the more pain they experience, which leads to poorer diet choices and worse sleep. The longer this cycle continues, the more severe the consequences (see flow chart below).

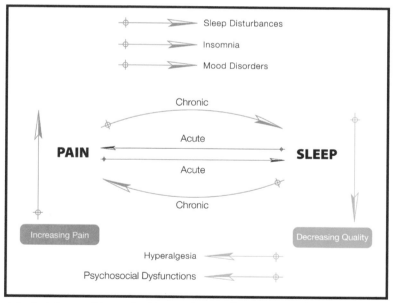

Adapted from: Olmos S. Airway Centered Dentistry: The A, B, C's of Treatment for Chronic Face/OSA and Closing Anterior Openbite without Ortho. Oral Health 8(3) | March 2017.

In addition, unaddressed breathing problems may result in chronic pain, and individuals who are suffering from persistent pain tend to have more acidic blood [74]. While not life-threatening, acidic blood cannot carry as much oxygen to the organs, resulting in more pain and poor sleep.

This cycle can be broken, fortunately, by changing the diet. Consuming less caffeine, and carbohydrates such as white sugar, wheat, potatoes, and flour, as well as carbonated drinks will help return the chemistry of the blood to normal. More vegetables, protein, and fruits as well as supplements such as alfalfa and green algae can help neutralize the pH of the blood as well.

Gluten, which can be found in wheat, rye, barley, and couscous, is associated with a serious condition known as celiac disease. People with this disease must avoid these grains, but even people who do not have celiac disease can suffer from headaches, digestive problems (such as bloating, abdominal pain, gas), chronic fatigue, tingling, weakness, and numbness [136–140] from eating gluten.

The oils in margarine, fried foods, and many packaged foods are harmful as well. Safflower oil, corn oil, sunflower oil, soybean oil, peanut oil, cottonseed oil, mayonnaise, and tartar sauce should also be avoided. While fats are necessary for proper hormone and nervous system function, fats from these sources are linked to chronic pain, fibromyalgia, arthritis, sinusitis, chronic fatigue syndrome, allergies, asthma, acne, flu-like symptoms, digestive conditions, endometriosis, menstrual cramps, Parkinson's disease, Alzheimer's disease, cancer, multiple sclerosis, heart disease, high blood pressure, depression, osteoporosis, pre-diabetes, diabetes … and the list goes on [141–147]. Good fats include oils from avocados, nuts, seeds, olives, flaxseed, and fish, and these should be woven into a balanced diet.

Not having enough of certain vitamins and minerals is

also linked to chronic pain or inflammation. Current research shows that patients with chronic muscular pain are often vitamin D deficient, and many who have obstructive sleep apnea are as well. Vitamin D, which is actually a hormone, helps to regulate calcium levels in the body. Calcium is important to nerve function and bone growth, which makes vitamin D very important. Supplementation with vitamin D should be considered, especially when adding calcium to the diet. Supplementing the diet with magnesium also helps reduce pain by restoring filters in the brainstem that decrease the transmission of pain signals in the central nervous system.

In addition, many people with chronic pain have problems with their digestion, or a condition referred to as "Leaky Gut." The protective lining of their stomach may be broken down, allowing inflammatory substances to enter their bloodstream and cause pain throughout the body. Supplementing the diet with probiotics (good healthy bacteria) can repair and restore the protective lining and stomach function. This, in turn, reduces inflammation in the body. Probiotics also help by blocking the growth of yeasts in the stomach that cause carbohydrate cravings.

Additional supplements that reduce inflammation include bromeliads, turmeric, and proteolytic enzymes. However, grape-seed extract may be the most powerful. Studies have shown that grape-seed extract can even help heal damaged cells in the nervous system [148].

In conclusion, a healthy diet should include:

- Green leafy vegetables – eaten daily for folic acid, calcium, and other vitamins.

- Vegetables – raw, steamed, or lightly cooked and eaten daily for an additional source of vitamins.
- Fresh fruits blended into smoothies with protein powder supplements to provide an excellent source of vitamins, minerals, and additional nutrients.
- Fish proteins, such as omega-3 fatty acids.
- Nuts – hazelnuts, raw almonds, cashews, macadamia nuts, and walnuts.
- Spices, such as turmeric, ginger, dill, garlic, oregano, fennel, coriander, red chili pepper, rosemary, kelp, basil, and sea salt.
- Salad dressing – should be made with balsamic vinegar, lemon juice, extra virgin olive oil, or mustard.
- Large amounts of water every day.

And should be low in:

- Yeasts.
- Most dairy products.
- Wheat.
- Red meat, eggs, and poultry.
- Sugars.
- Carbohydrates.
- Sodas and other caffeinated, sugary drinks.

Red meat, eggs, and poultry contain steroid chemicals that can hurt the immune system, as well as an inflammatory protein called arachidonic acid. Free-range eggs and poultry are healthier and have more beneficial fats and proteins. If eggs and poultry are eaten, free-range is preferred.

In addition to watching what you eat, it is important to watch how much you eat. You should eat moderate portions and stop when you feel full. Also, begin to exercise more if possible.

Diet may seem like a small thing, but following these instructions and changing your diet can improve the health of your entire body—including your airway.

CHAPTER 4

Case Studies in Obstructive Sleep Apnea Treatment

1: Male with sleep breathing disorder and pain and stiffness of the jaw joint

A young male patient presented with the following chief complaints: headaches, jaw pain, facial, eye, neck, and back pain. He also had the following sleep-related breathing symptoms: teeth grinding, crowded teeth, difficulty falling asleep, heavy snoring that disrupted the sleep of others, dry mouth upon awakening, morning hoarseness, and fatigue [69]. After an examination, his diagnosis was: severe cranial distortions (skull deformities), anteriorly positioned condyles (improperly positioned jaw joint socket), left middle turbinate pneumatization (an air pocket in the left middle nasal passage), and a severely deviated septum (the visible structure that divides the two nasal passages). He was also diagnosed with:

- a sleep breathing disorder
- bilateral capsulitis – pain and stiffness of the jaw joint

- facial/cervical myositis – painful damage of the facial and neck muscles

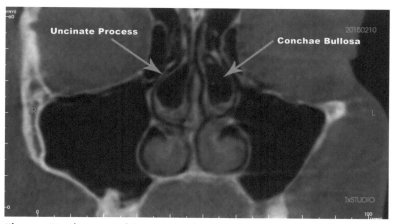

Figure 21 shows turbinate pneumatization (an air pocket in the nasal passage), which can compress the nasal cavity and prevent proper sinus drainage.
Adapted from: Olmos S. CBCT in the evaluation of airway minimizing orthodontic relapse. Orthodontic Prac. 2015.

He presented with posterior open bite (back teeth are separated and don't touch). This was the result of dental oral appliance therapy that did not resolve his chronic pain issues. This meant that after therapy to resolve his pain and headache complaints he would need orthopedic/orthodontic therapy to make all the teeth meet correctly.

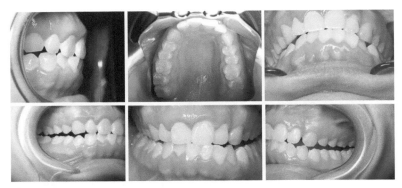

Figure 22

The treatment was divided into two parts. The first 12 weeks of treatment involved a combination of day and night decompression appliance therapy, NSAIDs, and a topical cream, a referral for a sleep study, MLS laser, trigger-point injections to the extension muscles, a referral to an ENT specialist for nasal surgery to correct the nasal obstructions, and dietary changes that included the consumption of protein, omega-3, grape-seed extract, and vitamin B, C, and D supplements, and vegetables with few carbohydrates [69].

After the initial treatment, the patient no longer experienced neck pain or headaches, and his jaw pain dramatically decreased, but he still suffered from severe obstructive sleep apnea. A second phase of treatment was started, which involved continued use of the day and night decompression appliances, the correction of his open bite, and the restoration of proper dental alignment. Specific orthodontic steps were also taken to restore the jaw joint to the optimal position in order to prevent airway collapse. Non-surgical orthopedic therapy (widening of the upper and lower jaws, and moving the upper teeth forward) were necessary to allow teeth to meet properly, and to increase nasal volume and breathing.

Prior to the treatment, the patient had a dramatically forward head posture that caused him to slouch, but this improved and the patient was slightly taller by the end of the treatment. Previous research shows that decompressing inflamed jaw joints through the use of oral appliances has been found to lengthen the upright position of the head by about 4.43 inches on average for patients between the ages of 13 to 74 [68].

Overall, the patient experienced significant improvements in his quality of life, his appearance positively changed, and he felt like a completely different person. He no longer suffered from headaches or facial, neck, and back pain, and his sleep disturbances stopped. Furthermore, his severe OSA was reduced to mild after he received treatment that decompressed his inflamed jaw joint and helped correct his nasal and oral malformations.

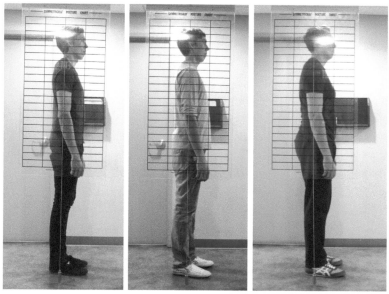

Figure 23

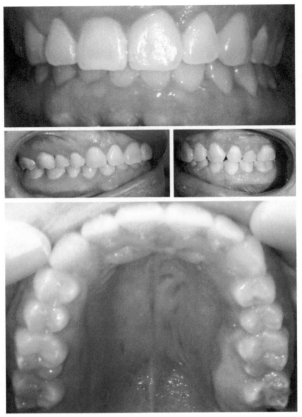

Figure 24

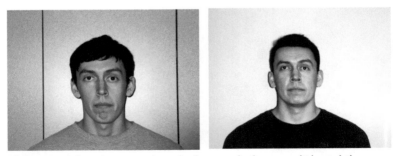

Figure 25. Visual comparison before and after nasal/dental therapy.
Source: Olmos SR. Orthodontic Practice (2017).

2: Expansion Therapy in an 11-year-old boy with moderate OSA

Expansion therapy was used for an 11-year-old boy who presented with moderate OSA based on a dental evaluation and a sleep study that showed the child had an apnea-hypopnea index (AHI) of 7.5 (Figures 22 and 23). Children are diagnosed with OSA if the AHI is greater than one.

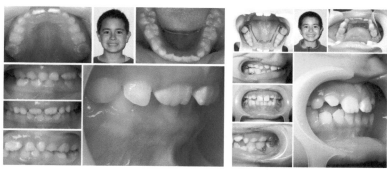

Figure 26   Figure 27

Figure 26 shows an 11-year-old boy who presented for orthodontic treatment. **Figure 27** shows the beginning of the expansion therapy. *Adapted from: Olmos S. Airway Centered Dentistry: The A, B, C's of Treatment for Chronic Face/OSA and Closing Anterior Open Bite without Ortho. Oral Health, March 2017; 8(3):44–56.*

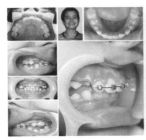 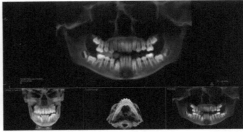

Figure 28   Figure 29

Figures 28 and 29 show the progression of the expansion therapy.
Adapted from: Olmos S. Airway Centered Dentistry: The A, B, C's of Treatment for Chronic Face/OSA and Closing Anterior Open Bite without Ortho. Oral Health, March 2017; 8(3):44–56.

After the expansion treatment, the patient's TM joints and nasal skeletal positioning were normal (Figures 26 and 27). However, pediatric OSA treatment requires reevaluation of breathing, which involves 3D mandibular correction through phonetic positioning to open the airway and prevent collapse (Figure 29). As this case study demonstrated improvement as a result of expansion therapy, it is recommended that all children receiving orthodontic treatment for dental crowding, an underdeveloped maxilla (upper jaw), open bite, and malocclusion (overbite) be evaluated by an SBD specialist [97].

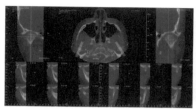 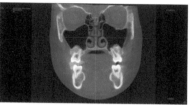

Figure 30   Figure 31

Figures 30 and 31 show the normal appearance of the TM joints and nasal skeletal positioning as a result of expansion therapy.

Adapted from: Olmos S. Airway Centered Dentistry: The A, B, C's of Treatment for Chronic Face/OSA and Closing Anterior Openbite without Ortho. Oral Health, March 2017; 8(3):44–56.

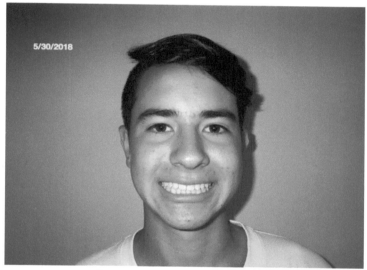

Figure 32 Here is the patient at the end of treatment who now does not have obstructive sleep apnea

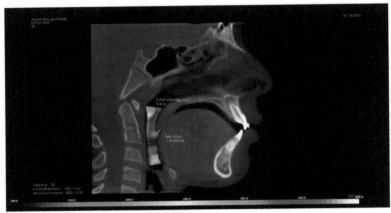

Figure 33 depicts phonetic positioning.
Adapted from: Olmos S. Airway Centered Dentistry: The A, B, C's of Treatment for Chronic Face/OSA and Closing Anterior Openbite without Ortho. Oral Health, March 2017; 8(3):44–56.

3: Identifying clinical signs and screening procedures for SBD in children and adolescents

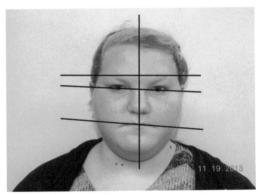

Figure 34 shows a patient with an uneven midline (canted plane of occlusion).
Adapted from: Olmos S. Airway Centered Dentistry: The A, B, C's of Treatment for Chronic Face/OSA and Closing Anterior Openbite without Ortho. Oral Health. March 2017; 8(3):44–56.

An additional case study emphasizes the need to identify clinical signs and screening procedures for sleep breathing disorders in children and adolescents [36]. This particular case demonstrated the elimination of OSA within three months through the use of Sibilant Phoneme Registration (phonetic positioning). This approach provides physicians with an alternative to CPAP therapy, which has been shown to intensify OSA by increasing midface deficiencies through the headgear effect [106].

In this case, the patient was 10 years old when she was referred for orthopedic development of a medical condition by a pediatric sleep specialist due to ineffective positive pressure and worsening OSA symptoms. She presented with a BMI (Body Mass Index) of 42.9 (morbidly obese). Obesity in children is a BMI of 22 or greater. In addition, she had hypertension (high blood pressure) of 130/112 for which she was taking an ACE inhibitor as well as metformin/Glucophage® for her type-2 diabetes. She also suffered from daily chronic headaches, facial pain (TMD), and bodily discomfort for which she was taking Tylenol®. Furthermore, she demonstrated a significant deviation from normal posture (Figures 30 and 31). However, her primary complaints at the time of the referral were dry mouth, sinus congestion, headaches, and frequent snoring. The patient was first diagnosed with severe OSA at the age of five. The results of her sleep study at the time of the initial evaluation were an AHI of 118 and her lowest level of blood oxygenation was 65%, when normal readings should have been between 98 and 100%. She was initially placed on CPAP, which she used for five years prior to being referred at the age of 10.

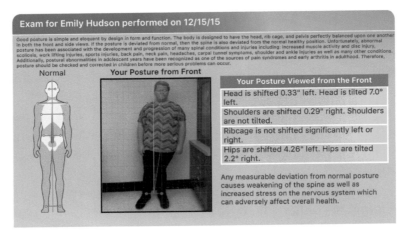

Figure 35

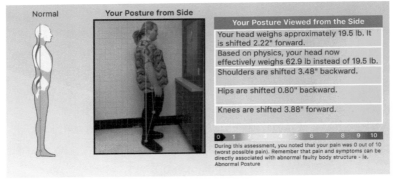

Figure 36

Figures 35 and 36 show the evaluation and quantification of the patient's posture.

Adapted from: Olmos S. Pediatric severe apnea/obesity/TMD/headache— Class III. Orthodontic Practice, 7(3) | June 2016.

At the time of the referral, it was determined that the patient's maxilla (upper jaw) was posteriorly positioned and deficient in all dimensions in relation to her skull. Therefore, 3D expansion therapy was the treatment plan, which included: 1) the expansion of the upper and lower jaw to increase nasal and oral volume, 2) reverse-pull mechanics to reposition the upper jaw and hinder airway collapse while simultaneously decompressing the TM joints, and 3) the use of a Tandem appliance to lever against the temporal fossa bones (sides of the skull) in order to facilitate the repositioning of the upper jaw. The types of appliances that were used are shown in Figures 32 through 35. The lower appliance was worn 24 hours a day, while the Tandem bow and elastics were used at night for 10 hours along with nasal delivery positive pressure (NCPAP).

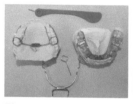 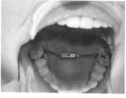 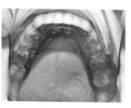

Figure 37   Figure 38   Figure 39

Figures 37-39 show the design for the patient's expansion therapy. *Adapted from: Olmos S. Pediatric severe apnea/obesity/TMD/headache—Class III. Orthodontic Practice, 7(3) | June 2016.*

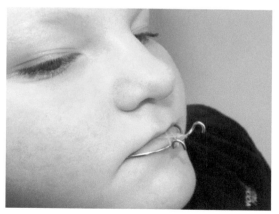

Figure 40. Lower appliance worn by the patient. *Adapted from: Olmos S. Pediatric severe apnea/obesity/TMD/headache—Class III. Orthodontic Practice, 7(3) | June 2016.*

After 4 weeks of treatment the patient's snoring and head-aches resolved by 100%; there was also a 50% reduction of dry mouth, and a 20% decrease of sinus congestion [63]. A dramatic uprighting of her posture was also observed, and this was attributed to increased nasal breathing and the reduction of TM joint inflammation (Figures 36 and 37) [68, 105, 149]. By week 8, improvement of her upper jaw position was ob-served, and her repeated sleep study demonstrated that her AHI decreased from 118 to 3.1. She no longer needed to be ventilated with her CPAP machine. The patient continued to show improvement of her posture and upper jaw reposition-ing at 12 weeks of treatment (Figure 37). Most importantly, the treatment resolved her sleep-related breathing condition. Overall, this case demonstrated that the dynamic skeletal de-velopment of a child with severe apnea could be improved upon through nonsurgical means with dramatic results [25].

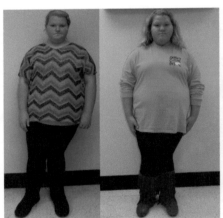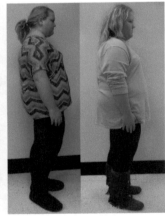

Figure 41. The images on the left (pink) were taken at the time of the referral, and the images on the right (blue) show the uprighting of the posture as a result of the therapy.
Adapted from: Olmos S. Pediatric severe apnea/obesity/TMD/headache—Class III. Orthodontic Practice, 7(3) | June 2016.

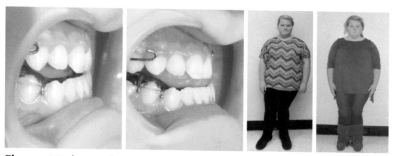

Figure 42 shows the progression of upper jaw repositioning from 8 weeks (left) to 12 weeks (far right) as well as continued improvement of posture.

Adapted from: Olmos S. Pediatric severe apnea/obesity/TMD/headache— Class III. Orthodontic Practice, 7(3) | June 2016.

References

1. Nieto J and Chair of the Department of Population Health Sciences at the University of Wisconsin School of Medicine and Public Health. The American Thoracic Society 2012 International Conference in San Francisco. May 20, 2012. San Francisco, CA.

2. Dement W, Vaughan C. The promise of sleep: A pioneer in sleep medicine explores the vital connection between health, happiness, and a good night's sleep. 1999, Delacorte, NY: Dell.

3. Kripke D, et al. Prevalence of sleep-disordered breathing in ages 40–64 years: A population-based survey. Sleep. 1997; 20(1):65–76.

4. Frost and Sullivan and American Academy of Sleep Medicine. Hidden health crisis costing America billions. 2016. http://www.aasmnet.org/Resources/pdf/sleep-apnea-economic-crisis.pdf.

5. U.S. Department of Health and Human Services. Healthy People 2010: Understanding and Improving Health. 2nd ed. 2000, Washington DC: U.S. Government Printing Office.

6. Peppard P, et al. Increased prevalence of sleep-disordered breathing in adults. American Journal of Epidemiology. 2013; 177(9):1006–1014.

7. Bradley T. Right and left ventricular functional impairment and sleep apnea. Clinics in Chest Medicine. 1992; 13(3):459–479.

8. Duchna H, et al. Vascular reactivity in obstructive sleep apnea syndrome. American Journal of Respiratory Critical Care Medicine. 2000; 161(1):187–191.

9. Guilleminault C, Connolly S, Winkle, R. Cardiac arrhythmia and conduction disturbances during sleep in 400 patients with sleep apnea syndrome. American Journal of Cardiology. 1983. 52(5):490–494.

10. Guilleminault C, Suzuki M. Sleep-related hemodynamics and hypertension with partial or complete upper airway obstruction during sleep. Sleep. 1992; 15 (6 Suppl.):S20–S24.

11. Palonmaki H. Snoring and the risk of ischemic brain infarction. Stroke. 1991; 22(8):1021–1025.

12. Partinen M, Guilleminault C. Daytime sleepiness and vascular morbidity at seven-year follow-up in obstructive sleep apnea patients. Chest. 1990; 97(1):27–32.

13. Kapor V, Strohl KP. Underdiagnosis of sleep apnea syndrome in U.S. communities. Sleep Breath. 2002; 6(2):49–54.

14. Simmons M, Clark G. The potentially harmful medical consequences of untreated sleep-disordered breathing: The evidence supporting brain damage. JADA. 2009; 140:536–542.

15. Levendowski D, et al. Prevalence of probable obstructive sleep apnea risk and severity in a population of dental patients. Sleep Breath. 2008; 12:308–309.

16. Okeson JP. Management of temporomandibular disorders and occlusion. 6th ed. 1994, UK: Elsevier Health Sciences.

17. Singh G, Olmos S. Use of sibilant phoneme registration protocol to prevent upper airway collapse in patients with TMD. Sleep Breath. 2007; 11(4):209–216.

18. Olmos S. Treating OSA and chronic facial pain (TMD): Keeping it simple. 2012, Oral Health. https://www.oralhealthgroup.com/features/treating-osa-and-chronic-facial-pain-tmd/.

19. Arens R, Marcus C. Pathophysiology of upper airway obstruction: A developmental perspective. Sleep. 2004; 1:997–1019.

20. Simmons J, Prehn R. Nocturnal bruxism as a protective mechanism against obstructive breathing during sleep. Sleep. 2008; 31:A199.

21. Mayer P, Heinzer R, Lavigne G. Sleep bruxism in respiratory medicine practice. Chest. 2016; 149(1):262–271.

22. Hollowell D, et al. Respiratory-related recruitment of the masseter: Response to hypercapnia and loading. Journal of Applied Physiology (1985). 1991; 70:2508–2513.

23. Gupta N, Goel N, Kumar R. Correlation of exhaled nitric oxide, nasal nitric oxide, and atopic status: A cross-sectional study in bronchial asthma and allergic rhinitis. Lung India. 2014; 31(4):342–347.

24. Grippaudo C, Paolantonio EG, Antonini G, et al. Association between oral habits, mouth breathing, and malocclusion. ACTA Otorhinolaryngologica Italica. 2016; 36(5):386–394.

25. Olmos S. Pediatric severe apnea/obesity/TMD/headache—Class III. Orthodontic Practice. June 2016; 7(3):10–14.

26. American College of Allergy, Asthma & Immunology. Allergy Facts. 2016; Arlington Heights, IL. Available at http://acaai.org/news/facts-statistics/allergies. Accessed February 22, 2017.

27. Centers for Disease Control and Prevention [CDC]. Allergies. 2011; Clifton Road, Atlanta, GA. Available at https://www.cdc.gov/healthcommunication/ToolsTemplates/EntertainmentEd/Tips/Allergies.html. Accessed February 22, 2017.

28. National Institutes of Health [NIH]. World asthma day: NIH research advances help people with asthma. 2011; Research Triangle Park, NC. Available at https://www.niehs.nih.gov/news/newsroom/releases/2011/may03/index.cfm. Accessed February 23, 2017.

29. Centers for Disease Control and Prevention [CDC]. Allergies and hay fever. 2016; Clifton Road, Atlanta, GA. Available at https://www.cdc.gov/nchs/fastats/allergies.htm. Accessed February 23, 2017.

30. Rothwell CJ, Madans JH, Gentleman JF. Summary Health Statistics for U.S. Adults: National Health Interview Survey, 2012. 2014; Hyattsville, MA. Available at https://www.cdc.gov/nchs/data/series/sr_10/sr10_260.pdf. Accessed February 24, 2017.

31. Ziska L, Knowlton K, Rogers C, Dalan D, Tierney N, Elder MA, Filley W, Shropshire J, Ford LB, Hedberg C, Fleetwood P, Hovanky KT, Kavanaugh T, Fulford G, Vrtis RF, Patz JA, Portnoy J, Coates F, Bielory L, Frenz D. Recent warming by latitude associated with increased length of ragweed pollen season in central North America. Proc Natl Acad Sci USA. 2011; 108(10):4248–4251.

32. Centers for Disease Control and Prevention. National Center for Health Statistics. National Health and Nutrition Examination Survey Data. 2002. Retrieved from https://www.cdc.gov/nchs/nhanes/index.htm.

33. Di Paolo C, D'Urso A, Papi P, Di Sabato F, Rosella D, Pompa G, Polimeni A. Temporomandibular Disorders and

Headache: A Retrospective Analysis of 1198 Patients. Pain Res Manag. 2017; 2017:3203027.

34. Abu-Arafeh I, Razak S, Sivaraman B, Graham C. Prevalence of headache and migraine in children and adolescents: a systematic review of population-based studies. Dev Med Child Neurol. 2010; 52(12):1088–1097.

35. Winner P. Pediatric and adolescent migraine. American Headache Society. 2012. Retrieved from https://americanheadachesociety.org/wp-content/uploads/2016/06/October_2012_Headache_Toolbox.pdf.

36. Carotenuto M, Guidetti V, Ruju F, Galli F, Tagliente FR, Pascotto A. Headache disorders as risk factors for sleep disturbances in school aged children. J Headache Pain. 2005; 6(4):268–270.

37. Rains JC, Poceta JS. Sleep and headache. Curr Treat Options Neurol. 2010; 12:15.

38. Smith MT, Wickwire EM, Grace EG, et al. Sleep disorders and their association with laboratory pain sensitivity in temporomandibular joint disorder. Sleep 2009; 32:779–790.

39. Sanders AE, Essick GK, Fillingim R, et al. Sleep apnea symptoms and risk of temporomandibular disorder: OPPERA cohort. J Dent Res. 2013; 92:70S–77S.

40. Olmos SR, Garcia-Godoy F, Hottel TL, Tran NQ. Headache and jaw locking comorbidity with daytime sleepiness. Am J Dent. 2016; 29(3):161–165.

41. Lam JC, Sharma SK, Lam B. Obstructive sleep apnoea: definitions, epidemiology & natural history. Indian J Med Res. 2010; 131:165–170.

42. Dieleman JL, Baral R, Birger BS. US spending on personal health care and public health, 1996–2013. JAMA. 2016; 316(24):2627–2646.

43. Gaskin DJ, Richard P. The economic costs of pain in the United States. J Pain. 2012; 13(8):715–24.

44. Express Scripts. A nation in pain: Focusing on U.S. opioid trends for treatment of short-term and long-term pain. 2014. Retrieved from http://lab.express-scripts.com/lab/publications/a-nation-in-pain.

45. Brandeis University PDMP Center of Excellence. The prescription drug abuse epidemic. 2013. Retrieved from http://www.pdmpexcellence.org/drug-abuseepidemic.

46. Horst OV, Cunha-Cruz J, Zhou L, et al. Prevalence of pain in the orofacial regions in patients visiting general dentists in the Northwest Practice-based Research Collaborative in Evidence-based Dentistry research network. J Am Dent Assoc. 2015; 146:721e3–728e3.

47. Levy P, Bonsignore MR, Eckel J. Sleep, sleep-disordered breathing and metabolic consequences. Eur Respir J. 2009; 34(1):243–260.

48. Lin YN, QY Li, Zhang XJ. Interaction between smoking and obstructive sleep apnea: Not just participants. Chin Med J (Engl). 2012; 125(17):3150–3156.

49. Alcohol and Sleep – Alcohol Alert No. 41-1998. National Institute on Alcohol Abuse and Alcoholism. 2000. U.S. Department of Health and Human Services.

50. Lu B, Budhiraja R, Parthasarathy S. Sedating medications and undiagnosed obstructive sleep apnea: Physician determinants and patient consequences. J Clin Sleep Med. 2005; 1(4):367–371.

51. Teodorescu M, Polomis DA, Hall SV, Teodorescu MC, Gangnon RE, Peterson AG, Xie A, Sorkness CA, Jarjour NN. Association of obstructive sleep apnea risk with asthma control in adults. Chest. 2010; 138(3):543–550.

52. Ruoff CM, Guilleminault C. Orthodontics and sleep-disordered breathing. Sleep Breath. 2012; 16(2):271–273.

53. Olmos S. Diagnosis and beyond. Sleep Diagnosis and Therapy. 2010; 5(2):14–16.

54. Marin JM, Agusti A, Villar I, Forner M, Nieto D, Carrizo SJ, Barbé F, Vicente E, Wei Y, Nieto FJ, Jelic S. Association between treated and untreated obstructive sleep apnea and risk of hypertension. JAMA. 2012; 307(20):2169–2176.

55. Peppard PE, Young T, Palta M, Skatrud J. Prospective study of the association between sleep-disordered breathing and hypertension. N Engl J Med. 2000; 342(19):1378–1384.

56. Marin JM, Carrizo SJ, Vicente E, Agusti AG. Long-term cardiovascular outcomes in men with obstructive sleep apnoea-hypopnoea with or without treatment with continuous positive airway pressure: an observational study. Lancet. 2005; 365(9464):1046–1053.

57. Aurora RN, Punjabi NM. Sleep Apnea and Metabolic Dysfunction: Cause or Co-Relation? Sleep Med Clin. 2007; 2(2):237–250.

58. Olmos S. CBCT in the evaluation of airway minimizing orthodontic relapse. Orthodontic Prac. 2015; 6(2):46–49.

59. Michels DS, Rodrigues AM, Nakanishi M, Sampaio AL, Venosa AR. Nasal involvement in obstructive sleep apnea syndrome. Int J Otolaryngol. 2014; 2014:717419.

60. Eccles R. Sympathetic control of nasal erectile tissue. Eur J Respir Dis Suppl. 1983; 128 (Pt. 1):150–154.

61. Akhter R, Morita M, Ekuni D, et al. Self-reported aural symptoms, headache and temporomandibular disorders in Japanese young adults. BMC Musculoskelet Disord. 2013; 14:58.

62. Olmos S. Chasing pain diagnosing and treating trigeminal neuralgia in dentistry. Dentaltown Magazine, January

2016; 34–40. Retrieved from http://www.dentaltown.com/Images/Dentaltown/magimages/0116/PAINpg34.pdf.

63. Simmons HC 3rd, Gibbs SJ. Anterior repositioning appliance therapy for TMJ disorders: specific symptoms relieved and relationship to disk status on MRI. Cranio. 2005; 23(2):89–99.

64. Motta L, Bachiega J, Guedes C, Laranja L, Bussadori S. 2011. Association between halitosis and mouth breathing in children. Clinics. 2011; 66(6):939–942.

65. Conti PB, Sakano E, de Oliveira Ribeiro MA, Schivinski CI, Ribeiro JD. Assessment of the body posture of mouth-breathing children and adolescents. J Pediatr (Rio J). 2011; 87(4):357–363.

66. Gagnon Y, Mayer P, Morisson F, Rompré PH, Lavigne GJ. Aggravation of respiratory disturbances by the use of an occlusal splint in apneic patients: a pilot study. Int J Prosthodont. 2004; 17(4):447–453.

67. Olmos SR, Kritz-Silverstein D, Halligan W, Silverstein ST. The effect of condyle fossa relationships on head posture. Cranio. 2005; 23(1):48–52.

68. Olmos S. Improving quality of life and faces nonsurgically. Orthodontic Practice. 2017; 8(3):36–42.

69. Cailliet R. Head and Face Pain Syndromes. 1992. Philadelphia, PA: F.A. Davis Company.

70. Hussain SF, Cloonan YK, et al. Association of self-reported nasal blockage with sleep-disordered breathing and excessive daytime sleepiness in Pakistani employed adults. Sleep Breathing. 2010; 14:345–351.

71. Vasconcelos BC, Barbosa LM, Barbalho JC, Araújo GM, Melo AR, Santos LA. Ear pruritus: a new otologic finding related to temporomandibular disorder. Gen Dent. 2016; 64(5):39–43.

72. Abrahams JJ, Glassberg RM. Dental disease: a frequently unrecognized cause of maxillary sinus abnormalities? AJR Am J Roentgenol. 1996; 166(5):1219–1223.

73. Olmos S. Dental sleep medicine & TMD: A system for Dx and Tx mini residency. 2017. TMJ & Sleep Therapy Research.

74. Lavigne G, Manzini C, Huynh NT. Sleep bruxism. In: Kryger MH, Roth T, Dement WC. Principles and practice of sleep medicine. St. Louis, MO: Elsevier Saunders. 2011; 1129–1139.

75. Salazar A, Duenas M, Mico JA, Ojeda B, Aguera-Oritz L, Cervilla JA, Failde I. Undiagnosed mood disorders and sleep disturbances in primary care patients with chronic musculoskeletal pain. Pain Med. 2013; 14:1416–1425.

76. Clinical digest. Pain and depression is linked to sleep disturbances in people with osteoarthritis. Nursing Standard. 2014; 29(8):16–17.

77. Brennan MJ, Lieberman JA. Sleep disturbance in patients with chronic pain: Effectively managing opioid analgesia to improve outcomes. Curr Med Res Opin. 2009; 25:1045–1055.

78. Snow JB, Wackym PA. Ballenger's otorhinolaryngology head and neck surgery. 17th ed. 2008. Pmph., USA.

79. Asthma and Allergy Foundation of America [AAFA]. Allergy research: Allergy facts and figures. 2017; Landover, MD. Available at http://www.aafa.org/page/allergy-facts.aspx. Accessed February 22, 2017.

80. Johansen P, Weiss A, Bünter A, Waeckerle-Men Y, Fettelschoss A, Odermatt B, Kündig TM. Clemastine causes immune suppression through inhibition of extracellular signal-regulated kinase-dependent proinflammatory cytokines. J Allergy Clin Immunol. 2011; 128(6):1286–1294.

81. Johansen P, Senti G, Maria Martínez Gómez J, Kündig TM. Medication with antihistamines impairs allergen-specific immunotherapy in mice. Clin Exp Allergy. 2008; 38(3):512–519.

82. Ubeda C, Pamer EG. Antibiotics, microbiota, and immune defense. Trends Immunol. 2012; 33(9):459–466.

83. Shea KM, Truckner RT, Weber RW, Peden DB. Climate change and allergic disease. J Allergy Clin Immunol. 2008; 122(3):443–453.

84. Cruz AA, Togias A. Upper airways reactions to cold air. Curr Allergy Asthma Rep. 2008; 8(2):111–117.

85. Shah R, Grammer LC. Chapter 1: An overview of allergens. Allergy Asthma Proc. 2012; 33 Suppl. 1:S2–5.

86. Roberts SD, Kapadia H, Greenlee G, Chen ML. Midfacial and dental changes associated with nasal positive airway pressure in children with obstructive sleep apnea and craniofacial conditions. J Clin Sleep Med. 2016; 12(4):469–475.

87. Olmos S. Appliance therapy. Appliance Therapy Group. Retrieved from https://www.ineedce.com.

88. Brown DT, Gaudet EL Jr. Temporomandibular disorder treatment outcomes: Second report of a large-scale prospective clinical study. J Craniomand Pract. 2002; 20(4):244–253.

89. Steed PA. The longevity of temporomandibular disorder improvements after active treatment modalities. J Craniomandib Pract. 2004; 22(2):110–114.

90. Bixler EO, Vgontzas AN, Lin HM, Liao D, Calhoun S, Vela-Bueno A, Fedok F, Vlasic V, Graff G. Sleep disordered breathing in children in a general population sample: prevalence and risk factors. Sleep. 2009; 32(6):731–736.

91. Li AM, So HK, Au CT, Ho C, Lau J, Ng SK, Abdullah VJ, Fok TF, Wing YK. Epidemiology of obstructive sleep

apnoea syndrome in Chinese children: a two-phase community study. Thorax. 2010; 65(11):991–997.

92. Pirelli P, Saponara M, Guilleminault C. Rapid maxillary expansion in children with obstructive sleep apnea syndrome. Sleep. 2004; 27(4):761–766.

93. Villa MP, Malagola C, Pagani J, Montesano M, Rizzoli A, Guilleminault C, Ronchetti R. Rapid maxillary expansion in children with obstructive sleep apnea syndrome: 12-month follow-up. Sleep Med. 2007; 8(2):128–134.

94. O'Brien LM, Holbrook CR, Mervis CB, Klaus CJ, Bruner JL, Raffield TJ, Rutherford J, Mehl RC, Wang M, Tuell A, Hume BC, Gozal D. Sleep and neurobehavioral characteristics of 5- to 7-year-old children with parentally reported symptoms of attention-deficit/hyperactivity disorder. Pediatrics. 2003; 111(3):554–563.

95. Olmos S. 3–D orthopedic development for pediatric obstructive sleep apnea (OSA). Orthodontic Practice. 2016; 7(2):24–29.

96. American Academy of Otolaryngology Head and Neck Surgery. Pediatric sleep disordered breathing/obstructive sleep apnea. 2017. Retrieved from http://www.entnet.org/content/pediatric-sleep-disordered-breathingobstructive-sleep-apnea.

97. Marcus CL, Brooks LJ, Draper KA, Gozal D, Halbower AC, Jones J, Schechter MS, Ward SD, Sheldon SH, Shiffman RN, Lehmann C, Spruyt K, American Academy of Pediatrics. Diagnosis and management of childhood obstructive sleep apnea syndrome. Pediatrics. 2012; 130(3):e714–e755.

98. Marino A, Ranieri R, Chiarotti F, et al. Rapid maxillary expansion in children with Obstructive Sleep Apnoea Syndrome (OSAS). Eur J Paediatr Dent. 2012; 13(1):57–63.

99. Usumez S, Işeri H, Orhan M, Basciftci FA. Effect of rapid maxillary expansion on nocturnal enuresis. Angle Orthod. 2003; 73(5):532–538.

100. Schütz-Fransson U, Kurol J. Rapid maxillary expansion effect on nocturnal enuresis in children: a follow-up study. Angle Orthod. 2008; 78(2):201–208.

101. Eichenberger M, Baumgartner. The impact of rapid palatal expansion on children's general health: A literature review. Eur J Paediatr Dent. 2014; 15(1):67–71.

102. Cerruto C, Di Vece L, Doldo T, Giovannetti A, Polimeni A, Goracci. A computerized photographic method to evaluate changes in head posture and scapular position following rapid palatal expansion: A pilot study. J Clin Pediatr Dent. 2012; 37(2):213–218.

103. McGuinness NJ, McDonald JP. Changes in natural head position observed immediately and one year after rapid maxillary expansion. Eur J Orthod. 2006; 28(2):126–134.

104. Rabago D, Zgierska A. Saline nasal irrigation for upper respiratory conditions. Am Fam Physician. 2009; 80(10):1117–1119.

105. Declet-Barreto J, Alcorn S, Natural Resources Defense Control. Sneezing and wheezing: How climate change could increase ragweed allergies, air pollution, and asthma. 2015; New York, NY. Retrieved from https://www.nrdc.org/sites/default/files/sneezing-report-2015.pdf.

106. Neck Surg. 2004; 12(1):9–13.

107. Papsin B, McTavish A. Saline nasal irrigation: Its role as an adjunct treatment. Can Fam Physician. 2003; 49:168–173.

108. Chirico G, Quartarone G, Mallefet P. Nasal congestion in infants and children: a literature review on efficacy and safety of non-pharmacological treatments. Minerva Pediatr. 2014; 66(6):549–557.

109. King D, Mitchell B, Williams CP, Spurling GK. Saline nasal irrigation for acute upper respiratory tract infections. Cochrane Database Syst Rev. 2015; (4):CD006821.

110. Georgitis JW. Nasal hyperthermia and simple irrigation for perennial rhinitis. Changes in inflammatory mediators. Chest. 1994; 106(5):1487–1492.

111. Rabago D, Guerard E, Bukstein D. Nasal irrigation for chronic sinus symptoms in patients with allergic rhinitis, asthma, and nasal polyposis: a hypothesis generating study. WMJ. 2008; 107(2):69–75.

112. Rama S, Ballentyne R, Hymes A. Science of Breath: A Practical Guide. 1998. Honesdale, PA: The Himalayan Institute Press.

113. Wingrave W. The nature of discharges and douches. The Lancet. 1902; 1373–1375.

114. Rabago D, Zgierska A, Peppard P, Bamber A. The prescribing patterns of Wisconsin family physicians surrounding saline nasal irrigation for upper respiratory conditions. WMJ. 2009; 108(3):145–150.

115. Zabner J, Seiler MP, Launspach JL, Karp PH, Kearney WR, Look DC, Smith JJ, Welsh MJ. The osmolyte xylitol reduces the salt concentration of airway surface liquid and may enhance bacterial killing. Proc Natl Acad Sci USA. 2000; 97(21):11614–11619.

116. Robinson M, Regnis JA, Bailey DL, King M, Bautivich G, Bye PT. Effect of hypertonic saline, amiloride, and cough on mucociliary clearance in patients with cystic fibrosis. Am J Respir Crit Care Med. 1996; 153:1503–1509.

117. Brown CL, Graham SM, Cable BB, Ozer EA, Taft PJ, Zabner J. Xylitol enhances bacterial killing in the rabbit maxillary sinus. Laryngoscope. 2004; 114(11):2021–2024.

118. Sengupta P. Health Impacts of Yoga and Pranayama: A State-of-the-Art Review. Int J Prev Med. 2012; 3(7):444–458.

119. Joshi LN, Joshi VD, Gokhale LV. Effect of short term 'Pranayam' practice on breathing rate and ventilator functions of lung. Indian J Physiol Pharmacol. 1992; 36:105–108.

120. Makwana K, Khirwadkar N, Gupta HC. Effect of short term yoga practice on ventilatory function tests. Indian J Physiol Pharmacol. 1988; 32:202–208.

121. Michalsen A, Grossman P, Acil A, Langhorst J, Ludtke R, Esch T, et al. Rapid stress reduction and anxiolysis among distressed women as a consequence of a three month intensive yoga program. Med Sci Monit. 2005; 11:555–561.

122. West J, Otte C, Geher K, Johnson J, Mohr DC. Effects of Hatha yoga and African dance on perceived stress, affect, and salivary cortisol. Ann Behav Med. 2004; 28:114–118.

123. Khatri D, Mathur KC, Gahlot S, Jain S, Agarwal RP. Effects of yoga and meditation on clinical and biochemical parameters of metabolic syndrome. Diabetes Res Clin Pract. 2007; 78:e9–e10.

124. Gokal R, Shillito L. Positive impact of yoga and pranayam on obesity, hypertension, blood sugar, and cholesterol: A pilot assessment. J Altern Complement Med. 2007; 13:1056–1057.

125. Bower JE, Woolery A, Sternlieb B, Garet D. Yoga for cancer patients and survivors. Cancer Control. 2005; 12:165–171.

126. Basso-Vanelli RP, Di Lorenzo VA, Labadessa IG, et al. Effects of Inspiratory Muscle Training and Calisthenics-and-Breathing Exercises in COPD with and without Respiratory Muscle Weakness. Respir Care. 2016; 61(1):50–60.

127. Hill K, Jenkins SC, Philippe DL, Shepherd KL, Hillman DR, Eastwood PR. Comparison of incremental and constant load tests of inspiratory muscle endurance in COPD. Eur Respir J. 2007; 30(3):479–486.

128. Patel AK, Cooper JS. Physiology, Bohr Effect. StatPearls [Internet]. https://www.ncbi.nlm.nih.gov/books/NBK526028/

129. McNicholas WT. The nose and OSA: variable nasal obstruction may be more important in pathophysiology than fixed obstruction. European Respiratory Journal 2008 32: 3-8

130. Schonhofer B, Franklin KA, Brunig H, Wehde H, Kohler D. Effect of nasal-valve dilation on obstructive sleep apnea. Chest. 2000 Sep;118:587-90.

131. Georgalas C. The role of the nose in snoring and obstructive sleep apnoea: an update. Eur Arch Otorhinolaryngol. 2011 Sep; 268(9): 1365–1373.

132. De Sousa Michels D, Silveira Rodrigues A, Nakanishi M, et al. Nasal Involvement in Obstructive Sleep Apnea Syndrome. International Journal of Otolaryngology vol. 2014, Article ID 717419, 8 pages.

133. Tikanto J, Pirila T. Effects of the Cottle's maneuver on the nasal valve as assessed by acoustic rhinometry. Am J Rhinol. 2007 Jul-Aug;21(4):456-9.

134. Cuccurullo S. Physical medicine and rehabilitation board review. 3rd ed. 2014. New York: NY. Demos Medical.

135. St-Onge MP, Roberts A, Shechter A, Choudhury AR. Fiber and saturated fat are associated with sleep arousals and slow wave sleep. J Clin Sleep Med. 2016; 12(1):19–24.

136. Hadjivassiliou M et al. Headache and CNS white matter abnormalities associated with gluten sensitivity. Neurology. 2001; 56:385–388.

137. Hadjivassiliou M et al. Gluten sensitivity as a neurological illness. J Neurol Neurosurg Psychiatry. 2002; 72:560–63.

138. Hadjivassiliou M et al. Neuropathy associated with gluten sensitivity. J Neurol Neurosurg Psych. 2006; 77:1262–1266.

139. Arnason JA et al. Do adults with high gliadin antibody concentrations have subclinical gluten intolerance? Gut. 1992; 33:194–197.

140. van Heel DA et al. Novel presentation of coeliac disease after following the Atkins' low carbohydrate diet. Gut. 2005; 54:1342.

141. Seaman DR. The diet-induced pro-inflammatory state: a cause of chronic pain and other degenerative diseases? J Manipulative Physiol Ther. 2002; 25(3):168–179.

142. Seaman DR. Nutritional considerations for inflammation and pain. In: Liebenson CL. Editor. Rehabilitation of the spine: A practitioner's manual. 2nd ed. Philadelphia: Lippincott Williams & Wilkins; 2006:728–740.

143. Cordain L. The paleodiet. New York: John Wiley & Sons; 2002.

144. Cordain L, Eaton SB, Sebastian A, et al. Origins and evolution of the Western diet: Health implications for the 21st century. Am J Clin Nutr. 2005; 81:341–354.

145. Simopoulos AP. Essential fatty acids in health and chronic disease. Am J Clin Nutr. 1999; 70 (3 Suppl.):560S–569S.

146. Simopoulos AP. Omega-3 fatty acids in inflammation and autoimmune diseases. J Am Coll Nutr. 2002; 21(6):495–505.

147. Cordain L. Cereal grains: humanity's double-edged sword. World Rev Nutr Diet. 1999; 84:19–73.

148. Cady RJ, Hirst JJ, Durham PL. Dietary grape seed polyphenols repress neuron and glia activation in trigeminal ganglion and trigeminal nucleus caudalis. Mol Pain. 2010; 6:91.

149. Tecco S, Festa F, Tete S, Longhi V, D'Attilio M. Changes in head posture after rapid maxillary expansion in mouth-breathing girls: a controlled study. Angle Orthod. 2005; 75(2):171–176.

CPSIA information can be obtained
at www.ICGtesting.com
Printed in the USA
BVHW021927250822
645478BV00001B/1